ALKALINE DIET FOR BEGINNERS

The complete guide to understand Alkaline Diet. Start the perfect meal plan to heal your body and eat well for weight loss

Meredith Loss

Table of Contents

This content is provided with the sole purpose of providing relevant information on a specific topic for which every reasonable effort has been made to ensure that it is both accurate and reasonable. Nevertheless, by purchasing this content you consent to the fact that the author, as well as the publisher, are in no way experts on the topics contained herein, regardless of any claims as such that may be made within. As such, any suggestions or recommendations that are made within are done so purely for entertainment value. It is recommended that you always consult a professional prior to undertaking any of the advice or techniques discussed within.

This is a legally binding declaration that is considered both valid and fair by both the Committee of Publishers Association and the American Bar Association and should be considered as legally binding within the United States. The reproduction, transmission, and duplication of any of the content found herein, including any specific or extended information will be done as an illegal act regardless of the end form the information ultimately takes. This includes copied versions of the work both physical, digital and audio unless express consent of the Publisher is provided beforehand. Any additional rights reserved.

Furthermore, the information that can be found within the pages described forthwith shall be considered both accurate and truthful when it comes to the recounting of facts. As such, any use, correct or incorrect, of the provided information will render the Publisher free of responsibility as to the actions taken outside of their direct purview. Regardless, there are zero scenarios where the original author or the Publisher can be deemed liable in any fashion for any damages or hardships that may result from any of the information discussed herein.

Additionally, the information in the following pages is intended only for informational purposes and should thus be thought of as universal. As befitting its nature, it is presented without assurance regarding its prolonged validity or interim quality. Trademarks that are mentioned are done without written consent and can in no way be considered an endorsement from the trademark holder.

Introduction

Thank you so much for purchasing the Alkaline diet for beginners the complete guide to understand the alkaline diet. Start the perfect meal plan to heal your body and eat well for weight loss. In this book, we are going to be talking about the alkaline diet and how it can help you to live a healthier lifestyle. Many people don't know this, but the alkaline diet has been pronounced to be one of the best diets to follow when it comes to better your health and wellness.

The great thing about the alkaline diet is that it works internally, alkaline diet helps you to change your body's pH level, which will change the way your body functions. Unfortunately, many people in North American countries have a very acidic environment, which can be extremely detrimental to their health. The alkaline diet helps people change their Ph. level and make them more alkaline. However, there's a technique to achieving the alkalinity levels. Which is what we are going to be talking about in this book, we will show you how to achieve optimal alkaline levels and how to maintain it the right way.

Also, we will show you the foods that you should and shouldn't eat when it comes to achieving overall health and wellness, especially when following the alkaline diet. With that being said, I hope you read this book very carefully as it is imperative that you do so. If you don't understand the information provided to you, then make sure that you keep reading it until you do. Making sure that you know every single information provided to you is crucial for your success with this diet, with that being said, let's get into the topic at hand.

Chapter 1: What is the alkaline diet and the history behind it

In this chapter, we're going to talk about the alkaline diet and the history behind it. Time and time again, many people have been looking towards following the right diet plan; most of the time, many diets cover the majority of the concern's consumer has. However, there has never been a diet which has managed to cover all of the issues people are looking to fix when it comes to health and wellness. Which is why the alkaline diet has been so popular in these days and age, the reason why this type of diet so well is because many people get what they want from this diet all of the issues have been addressed. Believe it or not, this is the only diet which reduces the risk of many diseases, but it also helps you to lose weight and to feel better overall. Making this diet one of the best nutrition plans to follow when it comes to seeing the results that you have been looking towards.

Many of you might be wondering what the alkaline diet is, we will get into that more specifically later on this chapter. But to give you a brief description on with the alkaline diet is, it is simply a diet where you are going to be consuming foods that are on the alkaline side which will cause you to say on the alkaline side. When you are on the alkaline side of the spectrum, you will be in a much healthy position when it comes to overall mental health and organ health. There is a scale from 0 to 14 which dictates how acidic or alkaline you are if you are zero on the scale that means you're extremely acidic whereas if you're on the 14th scale that means you're very alkaline. Best number to be at when it comes to following the alkaline diet and to see the most results would be to be around 7.5 pH level. The pH level 7.5 is one of the healthiest pH levels to be at, since it is a little bit more on the alkaline side but not too much. The pH level of basic water is around 6.8 pH, and our goal is to stay above the Baseline of the pH level and to be around 7.5 making us slight alkalinity.

One thing you need to understand is that we don't want to be in extreme spectrums of, either way, meaning that we should be more in the middle when it comes to being alkaline. There are many benefits to being alkaline, let's talk about that so you can understand it. When you are extremely alkaline, you will see benefits such as better digestion, better mental focus, better overall well-being, and finally, better physical performance. Many people don't understand the importance of you being on the alkaline side when you are alkaline, and everything gets a lot better when it comes to your physical health and wellness. Not only that, your mental focus will go up once you start to tip over more on the alkaline side. Naturally, our body wants us to be more on the alkaline side since being alkaline gives us a fighting power to fend off any diseases or illness. Most of the time, when people are facing disease such as cancer, their body is very acidic, which is why the cancer cells can survive.

Keep in mind that, if you take care of your body and become more alkaline, then the chances of surviving cancer will go up tremendously. Moreover, following the alkaline diet will also boost your immune system, which means that you will not even attract common cold and flu. this is one of the most powerful benefits when it comes to following the alkaline diet, and you will see benefits that will enhance your lifestyle. Now there are a couple of rules when following the alkaline diet, as you can tell the alkaline diet requires you to eat foods which are on the alkaline side. Which means any foods which are acid forming will be taken out of your diet. For example, when the following the alkaline diet, you're not allowed to eat foods such as red meat, any processed food such as sugar or any grains.

You are also not allowed to drink coffee, alcohol. These two drinks are very acid forming and cannot be good for you. One of the downfalls on following the alkaline diet would be that there's a lot of restrictions, you will be cutting out a lot of food which you might be eating for a very long time. This could make the alkaline diet quite difficult for beginners to start following. Moreover, the alkaline diet requires you to eat that way for a very long time. The alkaline diet is more of a lifestyle than it is a diet, many people who are looking to reap the benefits from the alkaline diet they need to make sure that they make it a lifestyle rather than a 12-week diet. For this diet to flourish in your body, you need to make sure that you are constantly eating good alkaline foods for a very long period so that you can see the benefits of the alkaline diet and therefore not see any negative benefits from the foods that you're eating. Which makes sense, if you really think about it. We should not make diets more of a one and done thing, and in fact, make it a lifestyle for us to see better health and wellness benefits from it.

If you are following a diet for 12 weeks, then you are not getting any benefit out of it, unless you are simply striving towards weight loss. Before we get into the types of food you should be eating when following the alkaline diet, let's talk about brief history. The alkaline diet was found way back in the 20th century. When a nutrition scientist began to test out certain foods on animals and to see where their pH levels are. The scientist noticed that when the animals were given more alkaline food, their pH level went up in their urine. Which was a great sign when it comes to finding out that certain foods can change your body composition and the way your body is functioning, fast forward to today this diet has taken off with many people who are looking towards bettering their health and wellness. Now the whole premises behind the alkaline diet is that you are not supposed to eat any food which is acidic, we will talk about that later on in this book. However, some of the great alkalizing foods would be, Lemon or any other organic vegetables and fruits that will help you to get more alkaline.

Making sure that you stay away from any food that has no process is very crucial one following the alkaline diet, which is why it is important that you understand what foods you should be eating and what foods you shouldn't be eating. Bear in mind that there are certain foods that you would consider alkaline, but they aren't there are many fruits that you should not be eating when following the alkaline diet simply because they're very acidic. We will talk about the fruits that you shouldn't eat later on in the chapters, however, please don't think that any food which is organic or natural is going to be alkaline that isn't the case at all. Many people tend to get confused, which is why you wanted to clear that out. The alkaline diet can be a very complicated diet if you don't know what you're doing or if you don't know, we will give you as much knowledge as possible on this topic so that you're ready to follow this diet.

When following the alkaline diet, you will essentially be a vegan. Since all meats are very acidic, you will not be eating any meat at all when following the alkaline diet. If you are someone who is already a vegan, then the alkaline diet will work very well for you. On the other hand, if you're someone who likes to eat meat and is looking towards benefiting from the alkaline diet, then you need to reconsider your priorities and fix it. The alkaline diet will work great for you especially if you have been in a very acidic environment, and you will see amazing results when it comes to your body feeling healthier and more rejuvenated once you start following the alkaline diet. Which goes for the meat eaters, once you give up the meet your body will thank yourself and therefore you will feel a lot better about yourself.

You have to understand that are or body is not meant to eat meat, the reason why our body isn't meant to eat meat is that we don't have the enzymes to digest it. Time and time again, many people think that they can get away from eating meat, or they feel like they're built a certain way that they can eat the meat. Keep in mind that we are all humans, and we all have the same digestive system. Our digestive system is not meant to digest meat; in fact, we are more of an herbivorous if you want to call it that. If being vegan is a problem for you, then the alkaline diet will not be the right choice. On the other hand, if you're someone who eats a lot of protein, regardless of where it's coming from then you need to fix it as well. Having a lot of protein when following the alkaline diet is also not a good thing since protein macronutrient is very acidic to digest, we need to limit the amount of protein that we're going to be eating. You still require a daily amount of protein to keep up with bodily functions.

However, we will have to limit the percentage of macronutrients on the calories coming from protein. You should not eat more than 40% of your daily calories coming for protein if your goal is to be alkaline. Even though we will be eating a lot of vegan protein, our body still does not need to have more than 40% of the macronutrients coming from protein. if you are in the fitness industry or you are looking to put on muscle, then there's a high chance that you will steer away from the alkaline diet. But let me reassure you that you don't need a lot of protein to put on muscle, thanks to online information many people have been misguided on how much protein they need to gain muscle and to achieve their goal. We do not need more than 30% of your daily calories coming from protein, which means if your goal is to put on muscle, then you can most definitely do that by eating lesser protein.

Many of the misconceptions you have when it comes to following any diet will be cleared up in this book, and truth be told you have been misguided when it comes to many of the things in regards to health and wellness. You don't need a lot of protein to put on muscle, are you don't need to have meat to put on muscle. Once you understand that, then you will be living a lot healthier life both internally and externally, and you will be thanking yourself later on in the years to come. The best way to explain the alkaline diet would be to take all the diets you have followed and combined it into one giant diet. Think of it this way, and it is like a hybrid of a vegan diet combined with the Mediterranean diet. this is one of the ways I like to think of the alkaline diet, and it is like a vegan Mediterranean diet without the wine, of course. If you have ever followed the Mediterranean diet, then you would know what I'm talking about. However, this diet was not popularized for better physical appearance or to put on more muscle; this diet was developed for people who are looking towards reducing the risk of cancer. As you know, cancerous cells like to live in a very acidic environment. Which is why the alkaline diet has been known to kill any cancer cells and diseases. Once your body becomes very alkaline, the cancer cells will not survive in it. This will make your body extremely resilient towards cancerous cells, and therefore make your body whole lot healthier internally and boost your immune system.

Not only that, but the alkaline diet has also shown to reduce the risk of blood pressure and to increase growth hormone, you can truly change your health, by changing your ph. levels. With that in mind, if you're someone who's looking to change how their body is feeling right now and to reduce the risk of inflammation or if you're someone who's looking towards putting on more muscle and to feel better about yourself and lose some weight then there's no better than the alkaline diet. Considering all the factors, the alkaline diet will also help you with better sexual performance. Many men who are facing issues with their sexual performance tend to be very acidic internally. Once they become alkaline, their body starts to feel a lot healthier, and therefore, their sexual performance goes up. Many people have claimed to improve their sex life simply by becoming more alkaline. The one thing you have to keep in mind when following the alkaline diet is that the number of macronutrients, you're getting into your body can dictate how acidic or alkaline you're going to be. Which is why it is imperative that you pick out the macronutrient needs appropriately, and of course, based on your goals. Many of you have a goal of getting rid of diseases, or to stay healthy overall. Which is great but one thing you have to keep in mind is that when following the alkaline diet is that you cannot have too much protein as it can become very acidic, on the other hand, you can't have zero protein since protein is a requirement for your daily needs. It doesn't matter if you want to put on muscle or to stay healthy, you need protein in your diet, which is why you can't get rid of it completely.

As you know, when following the alkaline diet, you are a vegan. Since you're not allowed to have any meat, you're going to have to resort to vegan protein to keep your body as alkaline as possible. When you are a vegan, the chances of you having too many carbs in your diet will go up tremendously. The reason why it will go up is that most of the foods that come from plants tend to be higher in the carbohydrates department. Which is why you need to make sure whatever it is that you're doing you are keeping your carbohydrates in control when following the alkaline diet. You also have to take into consideration the number of fats you're going to be consuming when following the alkaline diet, it is more so important that you get enough fats in your diet since it will help you with your bodily function and your hormone production. If you didn't know this, the amount of fats you get into your body is very crucial, and it is perhaps the essential macronutrient you can get into your body.

Our body produces hormones and other things thanks to the number of fats we're going to be consuming, which means you cannot neglect the amount of fat you are to be eating when following the alkaline diet. With that being said, you have to keep in mind that your macronutrient ratio will be a lot different depending on your goal. We are going to talk about all three goals which many people would be striving towards when following the alkaline diet. Most of the time, people following the alkaline diet are either looking to lose weight, be healthy overall, and not attract any diseases and finally to get rid of any diseases that they might be facing.

With that being said, we conclude this chapter, and I hope the chapter help you understand how the alkaline diet really works and how it can help you achieve your goal. If your goal is to live a healthy life and to see longevity, and better Sports Performance than this diet and genuinely hope you achieve it. The great thing about this diet is that it is so versatile when it comes to benefits, that this time I can work for anyone at any age. This guy truly is an all-around diet to follow and to make it a lifestyle, so if you haven't been pushed onto following the alkaline diet then keep reading as we will give you more reasons why you should be following the alkaline diet.

Chapter 2: Benefits of alkaline diet

The Alkaline diet has a lot of health benefits. Surprisingly, it has similar benefits to the top leading diet out there. Make sure you read them, allowing you to understand how this diet can help you in the long run.

Weight-loss in a healthy manner

As you know, there are many ways to lose weight. However, one of the most popular methods being used to lose weight is the Alkaline diet, and there is a big reason behind it. Many people don't know this, but Alkaline diet is perhaps the best way for someone to lose "body fat" instead of "body-weight." When following most diets, followers tend to lose a ton of weight, but most of the time it is muscle and water weight they are getting rid of.

On the other hand, the Alkaline diet makes you lose more body fat. Here is how it works, when you are eating right healthy foods for a prolonged period you have burned out all your glycogen stores, as your caloric intake drops. Which makes the body hit your reserves, and that of course, is your body fat. You will be burning more body fat, instead of muscle mass or glycogen, which makes it ideal for people looking to lose weight. Also, as you know, proper diet plays a huge role in affecting your hormones. Your insulin will flatline, and your growth hormone will go up, this will prime your body to burn body fat instead and will do so in a healthy manner.

Increased longevity

There have been many studies showings that the Alkaline diet can boost endurance. As you might know by now that alkaline diet can help you with cell rejuvenation or also known as autophagy, this process enables you to get rid of the old and weak cell and replace it with newer stronger ones. This process has shown to increase longevity and overall well-being, which is one of the reasons why the Alkaline diet can help you live a longer life. Moreover, some studies are showing that reducing calories in animals by 30% to 40% has shown to increase their lifespan. However, there is no study done on humans claiming such. Nonetheless, some studies are suggesting that monkeys that ate less food but more on the alkaline side lived longer.

However, there was another study indicating that it wasn't the case on 25-year-old long research done by another party.

Although there is no actual study backing these claims up, it does show that people who ate less had a fewer risk of diseases which could lead to longevity. Which is excellent news when looking at it from that angle, there is a lot of disease prevention that comes with the Alkaline diet, but we will talk about those later in this chapter. However, the main thing to remember would be the fact that Alkaline diet helps with autophagy, which enables you to rejuvenate cells, which makes it very evident that the Alkaline diet can help you with longevity and overall well-being, which is a great thing to consider.

Prevent diseases

There are many diseases present in today's day and age, and it very common to meet someone suffering from one. Which means, we need to figure out a way to reduce the risk of diseases for overall health and well-being. The alkaline diet has shown to lower risk of many diseases, and we will be discussing all the disorders the Alkaline diet can help get rid of. One of the many conditions Alkaline diet could help manage would be Alzheimer's and Parkinson's.

As you know, the Alkaline diet helps with boost brain health and to lower the risk of neurologic diseases. Some studies are showing that the Alkaline diet can help reduce the risk of depression, even though some people might not consider this a condition, it is still a significant issue in our society. The alkaline diet has also shown to reduce cholesterol, a 2010 study on overweight women found that the alkaline diet improved hosts of health complications including cholesterol levels (LDL) and blood pressure which is also known as the silent killer.

The Alkaline diet also helps with reducing type 2 diabetes, and there was one study done on men, which showed that Alkaline helped them stop insulin treatment. Although we don't recommend, you try this if you have type 2 diabetes, that goes to show you the power of the diet and insulin resistance.

Nonetheless, many studies are suggesting that the Alkaline diet can lower the risk of diabetes. Another devastating disease which alkaline diet helps getting rid of would be cancer. As you know, the Alkaline diet enables you to have a less hospitable environment for the cancer cells, which makes this diet an excellent idea for people who are looking to reduce this risk.

In regards to a healthier life, the Alkaline diet has also shown to reduce the risk of obesity. One study done on obese women suggested that alkaline diet reduced the risk of obesity in women, which makes sense as it helps you lose and manage body weight.

These facts about the Alkaline diet show you how the alkaline diet can help you get free of many diseases, and some have been backed up with detailed studies, whereas others are still being researched.

Nonetheless, you can't say that about other diets out there. The Alkaline diet will help you to get rid of many things and prevent you from further having any diseases. There is no better way of getting rid of illness or problems without the use of modern medicine, and this diet is so powerful that it will also boost your immune system which will help you avoid small issues like the common flu. All in all, there are many rejuvenating properties which come along with Alkaline diet, so don't overlook it and keep all the positives in mind before you look at the negatives.

Reduce stress and inflammation

The Alkaline diet has shown a significant reduction in inflammation. As you know, inflammation causes many chronic diseases such as Alzheimer's, dementia, obesity, diabetes, and much more. Now, there are many ways that the Alkaline diet helps you get rid of inflammation. The first one being autophagy, as you know alkaline diet helps you with cell rejuvenation cleans up itself by eating out the old self and rejuvenating them with the newer stronger ones. If your body does not regenerate itself with more new cells, the older ones have stayed for an extended period can cause inflammation.

Now that we've talked about many ways. Alkaline diet enables you to reduce inflammation; let's talk about how the alkaline diet can help you get rid of stress. You see, inflammation and stress go hand in hand. If you have high levels of inflammation, chances are your stress levels are going to be higher. Which means that if you lower your inflammation, you will reduce your stress levels, and as you know, this diet helps with better brain function. Alkaline diet enables you to send better signals to your brain, which would equal a better functioning brain.

When your mind is functioning at its absolute peak, your levels of stress drop down. Better brain function will also help you get rid of any stress you might be having and will give you overall better health can help you reduce weight. Overall, the health benefits you get from the alkaline diet will help you get rid of your stress or at least lower it. Which means, even if you are not facing any stress-related issues, the alkaline diet will help you have a better functioning brain and also help you get rid of any mental fog or stress you might be dealing. With that in mind, always make sure you consult a physician if you are noticing much more stress than you can handle, as it can be something severe and not fixable by the Alkaline diet.

Body detox and cell cleaned

Detoxing your body is very important when it comes to living a long healthy life, many people detox their body thru juice cleanse or other methods out there when the truth is that they don't work. Time and time again Alkaline diet has shown to help detox your body in both the cellular level and digestive level, which means the alkaline diet is a lot more superior when it comes to cleaning your body.

As you know, from a cellular level Alkaline diet detoxifies your body with the process of autophagy, what this process does it eat out the bad cells and replace it with healthier and much more stronger cells. Through this process, you will notice benefits such as a stronger immune system, prevention of diseases, and insulin sensitivity. It has also shown to reduce the risk of cancer, which is a great thing to know. Overall, this is how the Alkaline diet detoxifies your body from a cellular level. Let's talk about how Alkaline diet helps you detoxify from a digestive level standpoint.

People say that your gut is your second brain, and studies are showing how your stomach and mind are connected. Which means if your digestive system isn't functioning at its absolute peak, then chances are your brain won't either. It is essential to have your gut clean and working correctly, and this diet helps a lot with this process.

It has been shown that the Alkaline diet can help you clean out your gut and intestines getting rid of debris and junk. Sometimes, it is essential that we give your digestive system a break from eating all those "bad foods" regularly. Once you start your diet, your body will begin to slowly get rid of all the toxins present in your gut, and you see when you are eating all the junk food your body doesn't get a chance to clean itself.

Your body has to focus on digesting the food instead of cleaning out the toxins when you give your body a break from eating. It will start to clean out its gut, which makes this process great for people who have a lot of cleaning to do, but it will help you digest your food a lot better and also think better. The detoxifying body helps you tremendously with lowering the risk of diseases, which will help you live a longer life.

By now, you can see the pattern; Alkaline diet helps you from every single place to prevent diseases and many other complications. Which means there are more positives than negatives with the Alkaline diet, as we go along in this chapter, you will learn more benefits when it comes to Alkaline diet. However, remember that these will only work unless you do. You have to follow the Alkaline diet the right way to see these benefits. With that being said, I hope you have learned a lot from this book as we are just getting started. Now let's move on to another benefit.

Improved insulin sensitivity

As you know, the Alkaline diet helps you get more insulin sensitive, which allows you with many things. To understand it better, let me explain to you how insulin works. Every time you eat a meal, your insulin spikes up, then insulin is used to shuttle food either to muscle or your fat store.

When you have too much glycogen in your bloodstream, your body will send that energy to your fat stores. Whereas if you're insulin sensitive, your body will send the glycogen to muscle stores and will be used for energy. When you are insulin sensitive, you are more likely to use up all the glycogen from your food faster, and not requiring your glycogen to be converted into fats.

How Alkaline diet helps with curing insulin resistance is by using up all the glycogen stores, making your body use up fat stores and when you eat good food, it will use up all the glycogen and shuttle it straight to the muscle mass to be used for energy instead of being stored into fat. That is how the Alkaline diet helps you become more insulin sensitive; the benefits of being insulin sensitive are many. Once you become insulin sensitive, you will notice more mental energy and less mental fog, and you will also see less fat being stored in your body which makes it ideal for people looking to lose fat and or gain muscle.

Being insulin sensitive will also help you gain more muscle since most of the energy will be sent out to your muscle stores. It will be used to build stronger muscles instead of storing it into fat. Being insulin sensitive is a must, as it will also help you get rid of possible diseases such as type 2 diabetes. All in all, the Alkaline diet helps you tremendously with insulin sensitively, which will overall help you live a healthier life.

Increased production of neurotrophic growth factor

Believe it or not, the Alkaline diet affects your brain in a significant way. It all happens from the help of brain-derived neurotrophic growth factor, also known as (BDNF), this helps promote neuroplasticity. Neuroplasticity is your brain's ability to migrate and shapeshift, and this helps our brain to produce new brain cells. Once you have an ample supply of BDNF, we can preserve older cells while producing new brain cells. Which means your brain will be healthy and will keep growing because of the new cells coming. Multiple studies are showing that Alkaline diet to improve brain-derived neurotrophic growth factor, more specifically when it has to do with synapses, this is where your neurotransmitter travel cell to cell.

Diet has shown to promote this, and there was a study done where it showed diet following the 80/20 rule has shown to increase levels of brain-derived neurotrophic growth factor by around 50-400%. Now we know that diet helps promote (BDNF), more explicitly, diet helps when it comes down to synapses. It improves what is known as synaptic plasticity, and this helps modulate our moods better. For instance, we can strengthen a synapse or weaken a synapse. This process enables you to be in the moment when you need to be happy or scared; this will help you modulate that accordingly.

In layman's term, this process helps us change our mood and be reactive at the moment. For example, if you need to be more focused, you will be able to because you are modulating it. When your brain-derived neurotrophic growth factor increases, so do your (BDNF) expression. This process helps you produce more brain cells and protect more brain cells, and this affects your cells at a genetic level altering our DNA. Which makes diet one of the best ways to protect your brain, and this gives your mind all the help it needs to preserve and recycle out old cells.

Another thing which it helps with is producing more growth hormone, and there was a study done where it showed upwards of a 4000% increase in growth hormone levels. Which is huge when it comes to improvements, as you know, growth hormone is responsible for many things of them being weight loss. It is a plus to have higher amounts of growth hormone, in both men and women. I know that the information was very scientific, so to put in straightforward terms, your brain will rejuvenate a lot quicker.

It will also help you with controlling your moods, which will make it easy to adapt at the moment. Brain-derived neurotrophic growth factor will also help you produce higher levels of growth hormone and serotonin, which are both crucial for mental well-being. Overall, this makes Alkaline diet one of the best brains improving eating patterns out there. For readers looking for mental clarity and fewer moods swings throughout the day, Alkaline diet is your answer to all.

Boost immune system

There is a reason why having a healthy immune system is fundamental, as it will help you get less sick and be more "immune" to disease. The alkaline diet has shown to increase the immune system so we will talk about how it boosts the immune system. There was a study done on stem cells when it comes down to a diet individual; more specifically, they took a look at how the stem cells rejuvenated.

The study concluded that Alkaline diet depleted white blood cells, which is precisely what we want so our body can produce better and more efficient cells, which lead to more production of stem cells and lesser of white cells. Once you start to get rid of your old white blood cells, you will begin to produce new ones, which will overall help you recover faster. This study also found that there was a reduced amount of protein kinase A (PKA), which allows the stem cells to regenerate. If you have a lower amount of (PKA), this means that it will enable the cells to turn on the regeneration mode, which will allow them to create new cells.

As you know, the Alkaline diet has shown to reduce insulin levels, which is a great thing for someone looking to boost their immune system. There was a study done showing that high amounts of insulin levels, prevented "T" cells from doing its job effectively. The "T" cells are here to suppress inflammation and to fight off illness, "T" cells are most of the time responsible for getting rid of toxins which cause disease and inflammation. When your insulin levels are high, "T" cells are not performing at their highest potential, which causes our immune system to drop down.

When you are diet, there isn't a requirement for insulin spikes, which lets our body help the "T" cells work at a higher level and overall, boosting our immune system. Since you aren't eating foods which will spike your insulin a crazy amount, this will give your digestive system and organs a break. When you eat a big meal, around 70% of the blood and energy goes to your stomach to digest it. Which means when you are on a diet, you give your body a chance to recover. Everything is healing when you are on the Alkaline diet, which includes the digestive system. Meaning, your gut will be working a lot more effectively once you have given it some time to heal.

As you know, digestion plays a significant role in both our mental health and immune system, about 60% of our immune system is in our colon, which means when you are the diet, you are recovering your whole body and overall boosting your immune system. You will be doing yourself an excellent service if you can manage to boost your immune system, and with all the backed-up science showing how Alkaline diet can help you promote your immune system and reduce many other health problems, there is no reason not to start Alkaline diet as soon as possible.

More energy and muscle mass increased

Even if your goal isn't to put on more muscle, it is still good to have more muscle mass as it helps you with many things. However, the main thing having higher amounts of muscle mass helps you with would be a fat loss; having a higher muscle mass will help you burn more fat since it increases your metabolic rate. Don't worry, and you don't have to look like a bodybuilder for that to happen; nonetheless, it is essential to have the right amount of muscle mass, especially for women.

The Alkaline diet has shown to increase and preserve muscle mass, so let's talk about how that happens. There was a study done between two groups of men, one followed an 80/20 diet method, and the other followed a healthy eating pattern. Both groups followed the same workout but a different diet, one group which supported the 80/20 diet, which we will talk about later in this book, they noticed after eight weeks was, both the groups gained and preserved the same amount of muscle, but the group who were following the Alkaline diet lost more fat.

This shows that the Alkaline diet not only helped followers gain muscle and preserve it, but it also helped them lose fat simultaneously. The main reason behind that is growth hormone, as you know, the Alkaline diet has shown to increase growth hormone in our bodies. What growth hormone mainly does, it allows a lot less muscle breakdown and to burn more fat, which is one of the main reasons why the Alkaline diet is so beneficial for building and preserving muscle mass.

Another great benefit of the Alkaline diet as you know is higher energy levels, and there is a reason behind it. Many people know how it feels to have a sugar crash, you feel tired and lethargic, and the culprit behind it is insulin. When insulin is spiked up, your energy level goes down as this gives your brain a signal to relax. When you are an Alkaline diet, there are no insulin spikes throughout the day, which provides you with more energy.

Another reason why you have more energy when you are diet is that your body goes into a fight or flight response and since your body is eating food it was intended to eat in the first place, and our body produces more adrenaline throughout the day, which gives you more energy as you go along. Just be aware, at the beginning of your diet journey, you might feel less energized.

The reason behind it is because your body is still getting used to these changes, but after a week or two, you should start to notice more energy. Use the power to get more work done at work and gym. In my opinion, and this is the most significant benefit which comes along with the Alkaline diet. More energy makes you feel a lot better when you are looking towards making it thru those long days.

These are all the main benefits which come along when you start the diet, and the benefits genuinely outweigh all the negatives which might happen. These benefits can be life changing to most people, lowering the risk of diseases and increasing longevity it's a fantastic thing to have.

Chapter 3: How can the alkaline diet help you with getting rid of diseases

There have been many studies showings that Alkaline diet can help with reducing the risk of cancer, which is why this diet is one of the best things to follow when it comes to reducing the risk of any disease that you might be facing. Many studies are showing that most people who have cancer and start following the alkaline diet fought off cancer and started to live a healthy life. Which is why we always recommend that you follow the alkaline diet when it comes to reducing the risk of cancer, or if you already have cancer, you can follow this diet to get rid of it. However, if you are facing cancer, then make sure to consult your doctor before you make any abrupt decisions.

The reason why the Alkaline diet works so well when it comes to reducing the risk of cancer is it because it lowers your acidic level. When you have lower acidic levels, there's a less chance of your body attracting more foul bacteria in your body which will cause cancer. This environment will discourage any cancer surviving growth, which is why many people recommend you follow an alkaline diet. Some people might say the alkaline diet is not the right answer when it comes to reducing the risk of cancer, in fact, most people said as long as you eat healthy foods then you will reduce the risk of cancer. However, many studies are showing that your lung and your other organs might be higher in the acidic level, which is why you're attracting more cancer in your body. The main thing you need to understand when it comes to reducing the risk of cancer is that cancer likes to thrive on acidic levels.

If your body is very acidic, you will be in a higher risk of attracting cancer regardless, which is why the alkaline diet works so well at reducing the risk of cancer. Moreover, people have also shown to reduce the risk of inflammation, which makes it a great idea to follow the alkaline diet when it comes to reducing the risk of cancer. As you might or might not know, one of the main reasons why we attract cancer is the inflammation in our body. Many people get cancer because they are inflamed, and it's causing issues overall increasing the risk of cancer. Once people start losing the inflammation in the body, the risk of cancer lowers even further making it a great idea to start following the alkaline diet as the alkaline diet reduces the risk of cancer and inflammation in your body. Also, as you know, the alkaline diet has shown to rejuvenate our body. Once you start to break down your old cells and come out with new ones, your body will have more fighting power towards the cancerous cells.

Making the Alkaline diet one of the best diets to follow when it comes to reducing the risk of cancer. If your goal is to live a healthier life, then one of the main things you need to understand is your body recycling and detoxifying it very quickly. Which is where the alkaline diet comes on, any time you detoxify your body will be in much better shape to get rid of any diseases more specifically cancer. Anyhow, many people go on fasts and other things to detoxify the body. Which can also come in handy when it comes to reducing the risk of cancer, but the way these diet works is so perfectly that does not only detoxify your body but also makes it an alkaline environment where bacteria which because cancer cannot survive. Also, when you are eating these high Alkaline foods, you're not only making it better for yourself to reduce the risk of cancer. You are also making your body more bacteria-friendly, as you will be adding more good bacteria in your body, helping you fight off the harmful bacteria in your body. As you might know, we have two types of bacteria in our body, and we have the good ones and the bad ones. We ideally want good bacteria in your body, to fight off any disease that we might notice. Which means you need to make sure that you have good bacteria in your diet. As you know, the alkaline diet provides you with good bacteria and lots of it. However, it would be best if you made sure that when you have these good bacteria is in your body that you are drinking enough water to digest it and to keep your gut healthy.

Which is why it is essential that you drink more alkaline water, which we will talk about that later in this book. However, for now, you need to understand the importance of good bacteria in your body and reducing cancer, overall if your goals to minimize cancer and alkaline diet will provide you with that. However, if your goal is to reap all the benefits from the alkaline diet, then you need to make sure that a couple of things are in check before you do so. You need to make sure they get an ample amount of protein, fats, and carbs in your diet. As your diet will be very restricted when it comes to the food you are going to be eating, you need to make sure that you are eating the right macronutrients for your body. Which means, we need to make sure that you are eating foods which will give you a balanced macronutrient breakdown.

You will be eating no meat, which means you'll have to make up your protein needs are met through plant-based meals and plant-based products. We will give you some fantastic recipes to make good food. However, your goal is to understand that you are hitting the right number of calories for your required body fat on your goals. If you're not eating an ample amount of food, then your body will not have enough energy to fight off these diseases or problems. Which is why you need to understand how many calories you need and eat accordingly based on that. Some people are claiming that you need to be eating enough food regardless of how much or what type of food intake you are following, which means that it is more recommended that you eat enough food to get the optimal results. If you're going through chemotherapy, then you need to be making sure they are eating enough food regardless of what diet you are following. If you want to make sure that your chemotherapy goes successful, then it is crucial that you maintain your weight when you are going through this procedure.

There are some claims made that the alkaline diet will make it more successful for you when it comes to achieving chemotherapy success. However, many people are claiming this is entirely bogus. No claims are backing up that Alkaline diet helps with chemotherapy. However, many claims are suggesting that the alkaline diet will help you with reducing the risk of cancer and are getting rid of cancer entirely if you are following the diet. If you talk to your doctor, he or she will tell you that the alkaline diet is one of the best diets to follow when it comes to reducing the risk of cancer. However, this is not the popular answer for most people.

As many people have been brainwashed with media saying that alkaline diet is not the best way to go about, if the professionals are saying that the alkaline diet is a great idea, there's some truth behind that. To clarify, there have not been many studies claiming that the alkaline diet will ultimately help you get rid of cancer. Nonetheless, there have been many real-life situations where this diet has helped.

If you want to make sure that you are getting the best results possible, then make sure that you combine it with a good smoothie routine which will allow you to detoxify your body. It doesn't matter what diet you follow. If you aren't following the alkaline diet or your body is alkaline, then there's a high chance that you will not reduce the risk of cancer. Which means you will be in a much better position following the alkaline diet when it comes to reducing the risk of cancer, many professionals have claimed as such. One more thing to remember, if you're on acidic medications then you can counteract that with an alkaline diet. Make sure that the medicines that you're taking aren't going to disrupt your alkaline diet. We can't tell you which medicine will cause you to be acidic, the best way to understand which ones will is to ask your doctor.

To recap, the alkaline diet will help you keep your body at an alkaline level, which will allow no cancer or bacteria to start activating or to start forming. The alkaline diet will detoxify you and create new cells which will enable you to fight off cancer and make your immune system even stronger. Moreover, the alkaline diet will also help you with chemotherapy, as many people have said it will. Making this diet a no-brainer to follow. Just make sure that you are eating enough calories to maintain your body weight, especially if you are facing any cancerous diseases. I hope you understand how following the alkaline diet can help you with reducing the risk of cancer and many other diseases, to clarify there have been no studies showing that the alkaline diet will help you to get rid of cancer or any other sorts of diseases.

This has been a personal recommendation of many doctors, and an own review of many patients that the alkaline diet has helped them tremendously to reduce the risk of cancer or many other diseases. Which does make sense when you look at the benefits of the alkaline diet. If you're facing any of these diseases, then always consult with your doctor before you start any of this diet. Moreover, as always, know what type of medications you are taking and how can counterbalance your alkaline diet. Finally, truly understand what the alkaline diet is if you have to read this book a couple of times if you are feeling lost.

If you were going to follow this diet blindly, then it would be like riding a bicycle without training wheels. You need to understand the diet before you start following it, and feel it out before you can commit to it. If you can commit to this diet, then you will be in a great position in terms of seeing the benefits. One of the only problems with this diet would be the precise requirements. Also, you cannot drink alcohol or take any particular types of medication when following the alkaline diet. Make sure they have everything checked before you proceed to follow this diet. Once you have managed to do that, then you will be in a perfect position to start following this diet and to see the benefits of it.

Chapter 4: What are the different types of Ph levels test, and how to test them

Now that we have discussed the benefits which come along the alkaline diet, and also what the alkaline diet is. Let's talk about the next major issue, which would be the pH level. When following the alkaline diet, it is imperative that you have a clear idea of what the pH level is and what it calls for. Understanding how to test out your pH level, is very crucial when following the alkaline diet, especially in the beginning. To help you understand what PH level is, it is essentially a way to test out how acidic or alkaline you are. As mentioned previously, the scale goes from 1 to 14. If your pH level is at 1, then there's a high chance that you are extremely acidic. Whereas if your pH level goes to 14, that just means you are very alkaline. Ideally, you want to be somewhere around 7.5 pHs to see optimal results. Even when you are following the alkaline diet, you don't want to be in the extreme ends of either way. Meaning, it isn't always the best idea to be extremely alkaline. With that in mind, always remember to aim for a middle point in the pH level, which is 7.5. Your pH level will go up and down throughout the day, which is totally fine. However, if your average is at 7.5 pH throughout the whole day, then you should be totally fine and be at an alkaline state overall.

That being said, there are tons of ways to test your pH levels. The main two tests would be the saliva pH and the urine ph. Many people don't know this, but these two tests are very different from one another. One will be a lot more acidic, whereas the other one won't be as acidic when compared. Which is why it is essential that you understand the difference between the two methods and how you should use them accordingly based on your goals. The first thing you need to understand when it comes to pH levels is that the saliva will always be higher at the alkaline level. Depending on your diet, your saliva will be more readily available to see where your pH level is, based on the foods which you ate.

This will factor in the food you have eaten and how you have digested the food. One of the things you need to keep in mind when checking your saliva is that if you have eaten anything which is very Alkaline. If so, then it will show that your body is an Alkaline state, even if it isn't. This could be misleading when trying to find out if your body is alkaline. Which is why many people recommend testing your ph. level 30 to 40 minutes after you have eaten, especially when testing the saliva. Most of the time, your saliva will be the most accurate test when done correctly. Unlike your urine, your urine will be a lot more acidic nature and will be less alkaline when it comes to testing your ph. levels. There's a reason to that, the main reason why the alkaline levels will be a lot lower when testing out your urine is for a straightforward reason which is that your urine typically gets rid of toxins in your body. Especially in the morning when you wake up, and you haven't urinated in a long time, your body will be cleaning out all your organs and pissing out all the toxins which are available in your body. Which is why your urine will always be a lot more acidic level when compared to your saliva. Now when people are following the Alkaline diet, most of the time, they test both the urine level pH and their saliva level pH to get a better understanding of their body. You have to understand, when you are urinating, you are getting rid of toxins, which are most of the time very acidic.

Which is why you need to understand how to read your urine samples accordingly, your urine also contains a lot of sodium and waste products from all your organs, which is why specialist measure the pH level differently. The average pH level in urine is 6 pH, anything under 5 will be considered acidic. However, anything higher than 8 is alkaline. The same thing goes for the saliva pH levels, your level will fluctuate on how much food you're eating and what kind of foods you might have consumed recently. For example, a high protein meal before you test your pH level using the urine test will lead to a higher acidic level, which is why we recommend you wait it out. However, if you have a high alkaline level reading from your urine, there's a high chance that you might have thrown up a lot or you might have urinary tract infection. It is not ideal for you to be entirely alkaline when it comes to following this diet. If you are at the higher side of being alkaline from your urine test, then this could be not a good sign. You have to understand that you cannot be overly acidic or overly alkaline. Ideally, you want to be more on the alkaline side, which is why you need to be eating more alkaline foods to see better results as previously mentioned. However, your urine will always be on the acidic side, so be aware of that once you start following this diet. In fact, the water you drink is also going to dictate how acidic you are once you start following this diet.

Also, the pH level in the urine can vary differently. Many doctors don't even use urine pH level test your ph. levels anymore as it is so unreliable. The doctors will only use the urine pH level to understand more information if needed. Which is why we recommend that you don't use it either. However, if you're still stern on using this method, then there's a specific kit which you can get from any drugstore which will let you urinate in a box, and will test out your pH level accordingly. Since there a lot of methods to test it out, we're not going to get into all the ways of testing out your urine samples and your pH levels. Just make sure that you go to the drug store and figure out which one you want to go with, and then follow the instructions on the box.

This is if you actually want to test your ph. level using the urine samples, if you are eating the right amount of alkaline food then there are no worries when it comes to testing out urine levels and your pH levels overall. On the other hand, the spit or saliva pH level can be beneficial. When it comes to testing out your saliva levels of pH level, it is imperative that you understand how to use it correctly and how to get the best results out of it. You have to realize that the saliva level will be a lot more accurate when it comes to testing out your ph. level, as we told you previously saliva does not hold any of the toxicity which urine does. Most of the time, saliva gives you a better understanding of where your pH level is throughout the whole diet.

Your pH level should be around 6 to 8 when you're testing out your saliva levels. Ideally, your ph. the level should be at 7.5 as this will give you the best results. This is one of the best areas to be in when it comes to being alkaline. To test out, your saliva level it is very straightforward, simply go to your nearest drug store and get those strips which will allow you to get your pH level reading. The first thing you need to do is take the colored part on top off the strip and put it underneath your tongue, making sure you get enough saliva on it. Once you've gotten enough saliva in the strip then take it out after 30 seconds of putting it in your mouth and shake it up, it will give you a color scheme which will provide you with an idea where your pH level is. On the box of the strips, it will have the color scheme which will show you where your ph. level stands.

If you have ever used keto strips, then you will feel at home using the Ph. strips. Instead, it will test out your pH levels. One thing to make sure when you start your test of ph. levels using your saliva is to make sure that you haven't eaten or drunk any alkaline water before you test it. Give yourself at least 30 to 40 minutes before you start to use the ph. strip to see where your pH level is, as we previously told you whatever you eat will show up on the pH test.

Which is something you don't want; we want to understand where your pH level is at naturally in our body and not by the foods that we just recently ate. We know that the specific foods that we're going to be eating to alkalize your body are essential, however, once you do eat those alkaline foods, it will give you an unauthentic pH level reading. This sometimes happens after eating alkaline food, and your pH level tends to show up around 8 or 9, this would not be an accurate reading. Make sure when you do test out your pH level that it is correctly scheduled, and you haven't eaten in about 30 to 40 minutes this will give you the best reading when it comes to ph. level reading overall.

Now, the ideal urine and saliva pH sample should be around 7.2 when factored in both of their results. If you do both a urine sample and a saliva sample, and the average of both is 7.2 ph., then you are it the perfect spot. If your saliva sample goes below 7, then there's a high chance of your body starting to become acidic, add more alkaline foods which will allow you to become less acidic hence making you more alkaline. The recommended times you should be checking your pH level varies from person to person, and some people will say that you should check your pH level every two to three times a day.

However, some people recommend that you only need to check your pH level two to three times a week. We have found that the best schedule would be to test your pH level once a day, depending on how acidic or alkaline you are you might need to monitor it more frequently. The best way to go about testing your pH level would be to monitor it once a day. However, if you are more acidic and you're looking to become alkaline very quickly then we recommend that you check your saliva pH level two to three times a day to see where your levels are at for a week or two. Once you've achieved a right balance of pH levels, then it will be time to let it rest and then check your pH level less frequently allowing you to save money on strips and have a better idea on where your pH levels are.

Once you become alkaline and your body becomes more alkalized the chances of becoming acidic you are will drop. You see when you're more alkaline, your insulin levels will drop, your inflammation levels will fall, and you will notice less pain overall. Once you become more acidic, your digestion will slow down, and you will feel more pain, and your inflammation will go up. These are a great sign to see when you are acidic or when you are alkaline. Understand your body will give you signs, which is why we highly recommend you start understanding how your body functions when it is acidic and when it is alkaline. Just so you can understand a little bit better, the first thing you need to do is understand that the urine sample is to be you are used on a rare occasion or if you want to be extra meticulous with your pH level. Many doctors don't even recommend that you use urine to test out your pH level overall, as urine levels can be very unreliable when it comes to testing out your pH levels. Your saliva pH levels will be a lot more accurate, for the average person to test on how acidic or alkaline you are. If you are to test your saliva and your urine pH levels, then make sure that your ph. the level is at 7.2 which will make it the ideal pH level overall when it comes to making sure that you are at the alkaline side of the body.

As always, when you're testing your urine pH level that you test it after you have done urinating first thing in the morning, ideally midday when you have drunk enough water and your liver and other organs have been cleaned up. On the other hand, your saliva test should not be done once you have eaten anything, ideally. Wait for 30 to 40 minutes before you test your pH level after you're done eating food, as this could give you a wrong reading once you have eaten a portion of food and test your pH level right after.

The foods can dictate how your pH levels going to be, which is why it is ideal that you wait down a bit before you test out your pH levels. Furthermore, depending on your acidic levels, you also need to understand how your body functions when it is a lot more acidic, and when it is more alkaline. That way, you don't have to keep testing your pH levels, as you can tell by the way your body is performing to get a better idea of your acidic or alkaline levels. If you do eat alkaline or acidic food, make sure to counteract it by eating a different type of food to make sure that your pH level is balanced. With that in mind, now you've got a good idea on how to test your pH levels and the different types of pH levels when it comes to you being alkaline and acidic overall. You can now utilize the right methods, which you think will benefit you greatly, after reading this chapter. Make sure that you don't spend too much money on pH level strips, as it is essential that you don't take this very seriously. In the beginning, it is ideal that you test your ph. levels regularly.

However, once you have gotten the idea of how your body feels when it is acidic or alkaline, then you will not have to check it so frequently.

Chapter 5: Alkaline water and fruits

By now you have a clear idea of what the alkaline diet is, and you have most likely heard about the alkaline water and water can do in terms of benefits and making more alkaline overall. Many people say that the alkaline water can help you regulate your body's pH level, and prevent many diseases, including cancer. What is alkaline water, exactly? And why is it essential. When it comes to following the alkaline diet and getting better results overall. The alkaline water refers to its pH level, as you know, the pH level measure is house attic or alkaline you are the products which are alkaline or acidic. The scale ranges from 0 to 14, one being very acidic and 13 being very alkaline as we told you in the previous chapter with The Sweet Spot edges when it comes to being alkaline or acidic you should have a clear idea on how to work on it accordingly.

Simply put, the salty water has a higher level of pH level, which will help you regulate more drinking water hands, increasing her alkalizing level and will neutralize your acidic level in the body. Which is why tons of people recommend that you drink alkaline water, right after you drink or eating something which is highly acidic to counteract the balance issue and to alkalize your body overall. Fresh drinking water is generally around 7, where is the alkaline water is typically about 8 or 9 ph. each. However, the pH level isn't the most important things when it comes to making alkaline water. The salty water must contain alkaline minerals which will allow it to become higher in the antioxidants, hence making it more alkaline and change your body in a better way when it comes to alkalizing its body functions.

It isn't always necessary that the water should be higher in the alkaline level and cause any issues, it is essential that you make sure that your alkaline body is absorbing the minerals and making it more alkaline. Hopefully, that makes sense, make sure that your body is alkaline not because of the alkaline level in the food or drinks, but it is alkalize based on the inside. Although there have not been any studies showing that the alkaline diet can be right for you when it comes to making your body more alkaline, there have been some people saying that the alkaline water could make you get rid of many diseases even if you're not following the alkaline diet.

As you guys might know the tap water is not the safest when it comes to drinking, which is why many people who aren't following the alkaline diet and start drinking alkaline water tend to notice better health benefits because there aren't any added chemicals to it. Our tap water can be very polluted, which is why many people resort to bottled water or more specifically, alkaline water these days to see better health benefits.

Had our tap water been less polluted, we would not be drinking alkaline water to see better results. Just for reference, the tap water is around 7 pH or close to 7 pHs whereas the alkaline water has to be above 7 pHs to be called the alkaline water. Our bodies do a fantastic job of maintaining blood pH level, which is why it is not recommended by many people to start drinking alkaline water to see better results.

Nonetheless, alkaline water can help you alkalize your body quickly when compared to following and drinking normal tap water. If your goal is to become alkaline very quickly, alkaline water can help you tremendously as it is already alkalized and therefore will make your body more alkaline throughout the whole day once you start drinking it as we told you previously, if your very acidic and alkaline water can definitely help you become more alkaline. However, if you're not following the alkaline diet then it will be tough for you to become alkaline overall even if you are drinking alkaline water, so think of the alkaline water more as a supplement to your diet when compared to the whole idea behind it. Sure, the alkaline water will make you more alkaline to a certain degree, but it won't turn you into an alkaline body overall if you're not following the alkaline diet.

Alkaline water is not great just for the basic level, it is even better because of the mineral contents in it. As you know, the tap water does not have as many minerals as we think it does, more specifically, it isn't as clean and is less polluted when compared to alkaline water. Which is why most people tend to drink alkaline water, to see better results and to get more gains out of it. But once you do start drinking the alkaline water make sure that you are drinking it for the right reasons and that you don't have any health conditions, many people who do have kidney conditions or are taking medications to alter the kidney function it can be harmful to them.

Some of the minerals in alkaline water, cannot be healthy for most people if they are taking any medications or are working on some kidney rehab. Which is why it is essential that you ask your doctor before you start drinking alkaline water regularly, you see our body is not accustomed to alkaline water before we start drinking. Unfortunately, we are accustomed to tapping water and the normal water as we get in our country, which is why alkaline water needs to be assessed before you start drinking it for the right reasons. If your healthy male or female then you should have no problem with alkaline water as you'll see great benefits out of it, however, if you are taking any medications or under supervision make sure you consult with your doctor before you start drinking the alkaline water.

Since you have now understood the function of the alkaline water and how can help you accordingly, let's talk about some of the benefits that you might see from drinking alkalized water. One of the benefits that you will see from drinking alkaline water as a reduced risk of chronic diseases, more specifically, chronic acidosis. If you have a low-grade chronic acidosis then it might help you that you start drinking some of the alkalized water, the study has not been concreting yet, but there is some suggestion showing that it will help you. Another thing the alkaline water helps you with is to help you with improving your overall health.

As we know by now alkalizing your body will help you with better bodily functions, better digestion, etc. Which is why many people recommend they start drinking alkaline water to better yourself, however, you have to remember that if you want to see better results than you need to make sure that you are following the alkaline diet alongside with the drinking of you alkalize water. In fact, many people who are facing certain conditions should avoid excessive mineral intake, as mentioned to you previously if you have any kidney conditions then you need to make sure they discuss with their doctor before you start drinking any alkaline water. Another thing that the alkaline water can help you with is to improve athletic performance, again this study has not been concrete yet, but many athletes are suggesting that alkalize water has helped them perform for a longer period at their peak performance. If you're an athlete, then try out the alkaline water and see how it does for you.

Many people suggest that it will help you. However, many athletes say that it does not help them overall whereas some do so it is a gray matter and therefore needs to be found out by the person itself. Finally, there have been many studies showings that alkaline water can help you with digestion health. This is a great study, and it is up in the air, that the alkalized water does help you with digestion. As we told you previously when you're alkalized, your body will digest food a lot better, which is why many people start on the alkaline diet. So, it just makes sense if you are drinking alkalized water, that you will see better digestion health overall. Now, that you're aware of the alkaline water and how to use a properly let's talk about how to acquire alkaline water for the best results possible. One of the things you need to understand that is alkaline water can be very expensive once you start drinking it regularly, which is why we highly recommend that you make your own alkaline water.

If you have more funds to support your alkaline water needs, then, by all means, you can get your own alkalized water. We recommend Essentia, which is 9.5 on the pH level, this is the bottled water you get, which is alkalizing all ready for you. Make sure that you use this water if you are looking to get more alkalized water in your body, however, if your goal is to make your own alkaline water and there are some ways to go about it. The way most people do it, is that use normal tap water they boil it making sure that they get rid of any pollution in the water. Let the water cool down, then they will add minerals which they can easily find online that will make the water even more alkaline in fact adding lime juice will increase its alkalinity.

Once they have done that, it will separately put in bottled water and finally serve it when chilled. Utilizing this method will ensure they get rid of any pollutions in the water, and you will get a better pH level in the water as well. Your pH level should be around 9.2 to 9.5 if you use this method properly, giving you great alkalize water. However, you can live outside North American and European countries. Then there's a high chance that the water that you are getting from the tap is not drinkable, which is why you might have to spend a little bit more money on the alkaline water. Or you can buy machines which are known as water ionizer which will create alkaline water via called is ionization. This could be a great idea for people who are living outside of North America and European countries to get the cheapest water source of the alkaline water.

With that being said, this should help you really understand how the alkaline water truly works and how you can use it for your own benefit. Let's talk about alkaline fruits and how can help you when it comes to bettering your health. As you know, there are many alkaline fruits, as you can refer to the chapter in the book where the talk about the whole section of which fruits are alkaline and which aren't. You will get a better idea on which fruits will help your body even further, just like the water the alkaline fruits can truly help you with all the same benefits which the alkaline water can. In fact, once you combine the alkaline water alongside the alkaline fruits, you will see even better benefits when it comes to getting your body more alkaline and to see better health benefits overall. One of the great things about the alkaline fruits is that it always helps you with the bone density. It is crucial that you take care of your bone density as a can cause a lot of issues if you don't, truth be told since you won't be eating a lot of dairies when following the alkaline diet. Getting a certain amount of calcium and bone help will be diminishing down.

Which is why it is highly recommended that you take bone support, which will, in fact, come from the alkaline fruits are you going to be eating. Many of the alkaline fruits include blueberries, watermelons, grapes, etc. These fruits are known to help with bone density, which is why it is imperative that you eat these fruits when you're on the alkaline diet to see a better health benefit overall. Remember, the alkaline diet only works in a certain way if you are in conjunction with all the factors in. You have to make sure that your diet is perfect, you have to make sure that you are on the alkaline side in the beginning by using the alkaline strips and finally need to make sure that you are eating fruit to ensure that you are getting alkalized very quickly. With that being said, the take-home message from this chapter is that it doesn't matter if you drink the alkaline water or you eat the alkaline fruit, everything needs to be in proper conjunction when it comes to seeing better results overall.

You need to make sure that you are eating good foods 24/7, this will ensure that you are alkalis throughout the whole day and to really see the benefits of having the alkaline body overall. Use these tools as tools by itself, these tools will only accompany you with the alkaline diet. Don't think that these tools will only help you to get alkalized if you're not following the alkaline diet, everything needs to be proper if you want to make sure these things help you overall. Hopefully, you have understood the magnitude of these tools and how they can help you.

Chapter 6: How to make this diet your lifestyle

We will talk about what you should be doing, to make sure that you are not failing in your endeavors to start this diet to live a healthier life overall. This chapter will show you what you could be doing to make this diet your lifestyle and to not only help you to start the Alkaline diet and stay on track but also to live with this eating plan for the rest of your life. These daily patterns will help you to not fail on your diet, and we understand that you might fail a couple of times in any diet, and it is understandable to do so. Nonetheless, this chapter will show you how to make sure you are consistent and not failing. These habits have been followed by many successful people, to get optimal results in all of their aspects of life, whether it be fitness related or anything else. Make sure you start implementing all of these habits after you are done reading this book as it will help you to make this diet your lifestyle. The reason why this chapter might sound philosophical is that the only way you will see success with this diet is if you do it consistently. For you to do that, you need to change your current lifestyle by being more productive and disciplined. You have to remember, healthy eating is more than just a meal, it's a lifestyle.

Plan your day ahead

Planning your day ahead of time is crucial, not only does planning out your day help you be more prepared for your day moving forward, but it will also help you to become more aware of the things you shouldn't be doing, hence wasting your time.

Moreover, planning your day will truly help you with making the most out of your time, that being said, we will talk about two things 1. Benefits of planning out your day 2. How to go about planning out your day. So, without further ado, let us dive into the benefits of planning out your day.

It will help you prioritize:

Yes, planning out your day will help you prioritize a lot of things in your day to day life. You can allow time limits to the things you want to work on the most to least, for example, if you're going to write your book and you are super serious about it. Then you need a specific time limit every day in which you work on a task wholeheartedly without any worries of other things until the time is up. Then you move on to the next job in line, so when you schedule out your whole day, and you give yourself time limits, then you can prioritize your entire day. The same thing goes for your diet, make sure you allocate time for prepping your meals for the next day, which will allow you to have meals ready for you when you need it hence making it easy for you to continue on with your diet.

More focus on the task in hand:

This point is quite similar to the previous point, once you have started to plan out your day and you have become more aware of the things that you are about to do. With the time limit on all task that you do daily, it will create an urgency to get as much of the job done as you can before time is up and you are moving on to your next appointment. Which will help you be more focused on the task at hand and get more things done? Many people consider healthy eating to be time-consuming, which it isn't if you prioritize your time the right way. If you cook your meals the day before and you set times for your meal, then it should not be a problem.

Work-life balance:

You see, once you start planning out your whole day, you become more aware of your time and how to balance it out. Once you begin to write out your entire day ahead, you will know precisely what you are doing that day, so you don't have to do anything sporadically throughout the day. Always plan some time for yourself every day where you can wind down read a good book, meditate or maybe hang out with your friends and wind down. You will feel refreshed the next day, having to wind down and "chill out" will only make you a more productive person.

Planning out your whole day ahead will not only help you prioritize better. It will also help you be more focused on your task in hand and will help you have a better work-life balance. This also means that you are eating foods that you like once in a while; this will help you to stay motivated with the diet that you are following. So now that we have covered the benefits of planning out your day, let's dive into the how to's when it comes to planning out your day.

Summarize your normal day:

Now, before we start getting into planning out your whole day ahead, you need to realize that to plan your entire day, you need to know precisely what you are doing that day. Which means you need to write down every single thing you do on a typical day and write down the time you start and end, it needs to be detailed in terms of how long does it take for your transportation to get to work, etc.

Now after you have figured out your whole day, you can decide how to prioritize your day moving on could be cutting out a task that you don't require or shortening your time for a job that doesn't need that much time. After you have your priorities for the day, you can add pleasurable tasks into your day like hanging out with your friends, etc.

Arrange your day:

It is crucial that you arrange your day correctly, so the best way to organize your day is to make sure you get all your essential stuff done earlier in the day when your mind is fresh. After that's done, you can have some time for yourself to relax and do whatever it is that you want. But make sure you get all the things that need to be done before you can move on to free time for yourself. Another thing that will help you is to set time limits on each task, and once you start setting time limits, you will be more likely to get the job done.

Remove all the fluff:

So, what I mean by that is remove all the things that are holding you back from achieving your goals. Make sure you remove all of the things that are holding you back from getting the things that you need to be doing. If you have time for the fluff, do it if not, then work on your priorities first. In conclusion, planning out your day will help you tremendously! Make sure you plan out your day every day to ensure successful and accomplished days.

Be Grateful

We will be talking about how to be grateful and what are the benefits of being thankful for what you have! Now believe it or not being grateful every day will help you Get more things done while keeping your mood elevated, see when your thankful for the things you have you will start to feel like your mind will be in peace and joy. When your mind is in order and comfort, you will be more productive with all the tasks ahead of you that day. Being in a grateful state of mind will help you become less stressed and more positive, which will help your work quality by ten folds. So, it is pretty essential that you stay grateful not only for better work performance but to also be in a peaceful state of mind. This will also help you to do more positive things with your diet, such as eat clean through the day. Let's discuss the three main benefits of being thankful.

Helps you start your day:

Of course, if you start your day in a happy mood, you will more likely be keen to do more stuff and be more productive. If you read up on the most dedicated peoples and their day to day life, you will know that successful people tend to practice the same habits which I am going to be talking about in this chapter. The benefit of saying things you are grateful for, first thing in the morning will boost your positive vibes when you talk about the things, you're thankful for you will complain a lot less and attract negative vibes which is something we don't want! You always want to be in a positive mood as much as you can. To make sure you are in a positive vibe, write or say things you are grateful towards.

You will become more approachable:

Yes, being grateful will make you more approachable! Believe it or not, people do sense your "vibes" when you walk into the door. When you're more thankful about life, you are happier and more positive, which is what people want to be around. Who knows the next person you see could be an opportunity for you to grow your business or get a new job! So always make sure you are in a great mood and counting your blessings still, as good things will come to you.

Lowered stress levels:

I think this point is very self-explanatory, let me ask you this what most people are stressed about? Lack of resources plain and straightforward. A lack of resources creates 99% of the stress. Once you start counting what you have rather than what you don't have, you begin to become a lot less stressed, which is suitable for your physical and mental health! So, make sure you always stay in a grateful mood. If you want to learn more about how being grateful can change your life, I recommend reading "The Magic" by Rhonda Byrne.

So, all in all, being grateful will help you live a better life and be more successful. Now you might be wondering how to be thankful throughout the day since it is so hard to block out ungrateful thoughts, well I'll show you three techniques that will help you combat your ungrateful thoughts and keep you in a grateful "vibe" most of your life.

Write ten things you are grateful for every morning:

You see, writing what you are thankful for will make your life a lot easier and help you start your day in gratitude. What I want you to do is first get a notebook/diary, then as soon as you wake up, I want you to write ten things you're grateful for. This could be anything from small as having water to drink to have a nice car, the whole point of it is to make you start your day in gratitude as the way you start your day is the way your entire day is going to be most of the time. So, make sure to start your day on the right foot by writing down ten things you're grateful towards.

Don't forget the 1:5 ratio:

This is something I thought about, and it works great for me, you see whenever I say something I am angry or not grateful for I always say five things I am super thankful for right after to get myself into the grateful "vibe" in the beginning this method will be your best friend as it will save you from killing your "vibe".

Cut out negative people:

This task might be the hardest to do, but it is quite essential, see the people who you are around are the people who will create your personality. So if you are around negative people, you will develop adverse circumstances for yourself, so if you are around people who are not upbeat about life and find everything wrong and never see the good in anyone, you need to cut them out and be around people who are happy and ready for what life has to offer. Now I get it, some cynical people can be your family members, and you can't get rid of them, the best thing to do is 1. Make them understand what they are doing wrong 2. Show them how they can make their life better and if they still want to remain the same, then keep your distance.

In conclusion, it is essential that you are in a grateful "vibe" as it will not only help you with your mental and physical health, but it will also help you attract better people and better circumstances. Don't forget to practice the three methods we discussed in this chapter for you to be in a grateful 'vibe" throughout the day and life! That being said I hope this chapter shed some light on the importance of being grateful and how it can make or break your life, and I hope you don't take this chapter lightly being grateful is the most critical thing you can do to turn your life around. So be thankful!

Now that we have covered the part of being grateful, and how it can help you with your day to day life and eating habits. Let us give you some concrete ideas on how to change the way you live your experience and to make it better.

Stop multitasking

I think we are all guilty of this at a time, and if are multitasking right now, I need you to stop. Now multitasking could be a lot of things, it could be as small as cooking and texting at the same time, or it could be as big as working on two projects at the same time. Studies are showing how multitasking can reduce your quality of work, which something you don't want to do if your goal is to get the best result out of the thing that you are doing. That being said, there are a lot more reasons as to why you shouldn't be multitasking, so without further ado, lets dive into the primary reasons why multitasking can be harmful.

You're not as productive.

Believe it or not, you tend to be a lot less productive when you are multitasking. When you go from one project to another or anything else for that matter, you don't put all your effort into your work. You are always worried about the project that you will be moving into next. So, moving back and forth from one project to another will definitely affect your productivity if you want to get the most out of your work you need to be focused on one thing at a time and make sure you get it done to the best of your abilities. Plus, you are more likely to make mistakes, which will not help you work at the best of your ability.

You become slower at your work.

When you are multitasking, chances are you will end up being slower at completing your projects. You would be in a better position if you were to focus on one project at a time instead of going back and forth, which of course helps you complete them faster. So, the thing that enables you to be faster at your projects when you're not multitasking is the mindset, we often don't realize how much mindset comes into play. When you are going back and forth from one project to another, you are in a different mental state going into another project which takes time to build and break. So, by the time you have managed to get into the mindset of project A you are already moving into project B, it is always best that you devote your time and energy one project at a time if you want it to doe did an at a faster pace.

Affects your creativity

This is a significant disadvantage of multitasking, and studies are showing that multitasking can negatively affect your creativity. When something requires too much focus from your end, it becomes harmful to your creativity, and you need a lot more attention when multitasking compared to working on one thing at a time. If you want to succeed and live a better life, then you need to be creative, so if multitasking affects your creativity, then you need to stop doing that.

By now, you can see how multitasking can hinder the ability for you to work at your best. These three things listed above are a no-no when it comes to living a better and more productive life; not only does multitasking help not be prolific but makes you slower and less creative. So, all the benefits you thought you were getting multitasking was not accurate after all, nonetheless, by now, you might be wondering how to go about working most efficiently. Well, the best way to put it is to work on one project at a time, I want you to put all your time and energy in the project you are doing currently and not worry about other projects. Make sure you set yourself goals when you start the project which will help you be more efficient and faster at your work, so an example would be "you will not move on to another project until project A has been completed" or you have managed to hit a certain threshold at that specific project. So, to sum it all up.

Do one project at a time

Don't move on until it is completed or you have managed to hit a certain threshold.

Set yourself a goal (time, quality, etc.)

All in all, multitasking will do you no good. It will only make you slower at your work and make you less productive. Making sure you stop multitasking is essential, as it will only help you live a better life. One thing to remember from this chapter is to put all your energy at one thing at a time, and this will yield you a lot of better projects or anything that you are working towards to be great. If you want to be more successful and live a better life, you need to make sure your projects are quality as I can't stress this point enough. You are probably reading this book because you want to get better at living your life or achieve goals that you just haven't yet, one of the reasons why you are not living the life that you want or haven't reached your goal could be a lot of things but, one of the items could be the quality of your work which could be taking a hit because of you multitasking. So, review yourself, and find out why you haven't achieved your goal and why you are not living the life that you want.

Then if you happen to stumble upon multitasking being the limiting factor or the quality of your work, I want you to stop multitasking and start working on one project at a time while giving it your full attention. What you will notice is that your work will have a higher quality and will be completed in a quicker amount of time following the steps listed above, which will change your life and help you achieve your life goals in a better more efficient way.

After reading this chapter, many might be thinking that this is more of a self-help book than it is a diet book. The Truth is that we want you to understand how to live a better life by changing the habits that you are currently following. Truth be told, following a diet and making it a lifestyle is a lot more work than you think it is. For you to make it easy, you need to understand that you need to change your habits in order to be successful at this diet, which means you need to change the way you move the way you think and the way you perform.

This chapter gives you a clear idea on how to start living a better life by changing up your habits, once you do change your practices you will notice that following the Alkaline diet as a whole will be very easy for you. The reason why it will be straightforward for you is that you will change the way you move and the change the way you live your life in general. Changing the way you live your life will not only help you get better results, but it will also help you to follow this diet as a lifestyle, many people confuse diet as not being a part of a lifestyle, and it is something that they're supporting to better their health.

But the truth is that when they're following a diet, they don't realize that it needs to be a lifestyle for it to be a health benefit, if you want to be healthier then you need to make sure that you're taking care of your health 24/7 365 days a year. Which means you need to make this a lifestyle, and for you to make this a lifestyle, we need to understand some self-help techniques to keep it sustained for a more extended period. Which is why this chapter is more self-help oriented, we wanted to make sure that this book is different than any other books that you've read when it comes to following the Alkaline diet. The way we're going to be delivering it is by showing you how to change your lifestyle for the better instead of the worst. We're not just going to give you foods to eat and how to follow the Alkaline diet, but in fact, we're going to change the way you eat overall and to make it a better experience for you once you start getting into this diet. With that being said, I hope this chapter was helpful to you, and we will see you in the next chapter.

Chapter 7: Working out and alkaline diet

In this chapter, we will talk about sets-reps-temp-rest, and we will also touch upon resistance training and what it entails. Knowing the basics is essential before you start any workout plan or try and understand anything, you need to understand what this portion of the book entails. Meaning, you need to know the basics, and you need to know all the primal movements. We are making you more knowledgeable with working out so you have a better idea on how to program workouts yourself. Keep in mind that having a good workout plan alongside your alkaline diet is very important. Which is why we are heavily educating you on the topic of working out. Without further ado, let's get into it.

You know how resistance training can be beneficial for anyone. Whether you want to put on muscle, lose fat or to stay in shape, it is crucial that you have resistance training in your program. Now let us get into the specifics of what resistance training is and why you should be using it, resistance training in layman's term is a form or a type of exercise that you use for muscular strength and endurance. Now let's get into the whys, if your goal is to put on muscle you need to achieve micro tears for your muscle to grow stronger and more significant, this process is called hypertrophy. Resistance training will also help if your goal is to get in shape or lose weight while having a considerable amount of muscle fibers, which will raise your metabolism and will help you burn more energy at rest, meaning fat and glycogen. If you're a fifty-year-old women who just want to stay in shape resistance training will help you gain strength, Now hypothetically speaking, if you were to trip over and fall with no one around to help you get back up on your feet, you need strength to push yourself up off the floor, when you are young that's the last thing you are worried about but as you get older something as easy as this could be a struggle. If you can't get yourself up off the floor and no one is there to help you. Guess what you're in trouble, and the sooner you start working on your strength, the better. That doesn't mean you need to train like a bodybuilder you need to do some type of resistance training to stay at an optimal health level. I will be giving an example workout plan in the following chapters.

Now let us talk about resistance training for people looking to put on muscle. For someone who is trying to put on as much muscle as possible more volume is the key, usually. After a workout, the normal human being will recover from it in about forty-eight to seventy-two hours. That is depending on stress, sleep, nutrition, genetics but the average time is forty-eight to seventy-two hours to recover from a workout. If you have gone online and looked up workout programs for bodybuilding most of them are one to two body part split, and you only train the muscle group once a week, that's hundred and sixty-eight hours you have not trained that specific muscle. The conclusion is that you can train a particular muscle multiple times a week, which means you will put on more muscle and get stronger quicker than someone who only trains that specific muscle once a week. Your workouts are is going to be more than one body part a day unlike a bodybuilding split and should be repeated couple of times a week for someone who has the time for it. Three to five times a week would be perfect for them to achieve their goals in terms of putting on muscle if you don't have the time for it a full body workout three times a week with higher intensity (heavier weights) can be used to yield similar effects. The man focus here is to train those muscles every two to four days making sure we are fully recovered first.

Now, for someone who is in their mid-fifties trying to get in shape because your doctor told you to or you have decided to embark on this journey yourself. Then the resistance training part will be a lot more different for you than someone who is just trying to get bigger and muscular, our primary focus for someone who wants to stay healthy and get in shape is to gain strength, start firing muscles that we have not used before and started putting on some muscle so we can actually achieve the first two things listed here. For people with the needs listed above the best way to get to your goals will be full body training meaning all your major muscles in one day, don't worry doesn't take longer than one hour to do so. You should perform these workouts three times in a week, primary goal for this is to make sure we are using slow tempo meaning we are gradually performing the exercise and making sure we are actually firing the right muscle fiber, at first it would seem like it's hard to actually fire the exact muscles you are trying to fire. But if you consciously think about that muscle to "fire" eventually you will start to feel it, that is if your form is correct. Take your time with your technique first. Don't overlook it. That goes for anyone.

Sets, Repetition, Tempo, Rest

Let me explain to you what exactly, sets, repetition tempo is. Sets- how many times you perform an exercise before moving on to the next exercise. Repetition- How many times continuously you perform the exercises without any break. Tempo- How fast or slow you perform a rep. Rest- How long you take between sets to start another working set. These four components are the single most important aspects of your training. You need to make sure you are actually following the rest set and tempo according to your training age, and your goals. If someone is in peak health and is an experienced trainee, then I would not make him wait five minutes before we get into our next set, unless we are training heavy or going to attempt a one rep max if that's the case then rest till we are fully recovered before going into the exercise.

Another thing that factors in when it comes to the three components is what your goals are and what type of training you are into or following right now. If your goal is to get lean and build up your cardiovascular health, then shorter breaks with a fast tempo and with a couple of sets will work better for you to yield those results. Whereas when we look at a different spectrum if your goal is put on the most muscle as possible, then time under tension is the key, meaning that we will have to slow down the tempo and make the rest in between longer and do multiple sets of the exercise to yield those results. There is no cookie cutter rest, sets, a tempo that will do for any type of workout. People who have been training for a while tend to need a lot less rest in between than someone who is just starting to exercise since it's a new stimulus for them.

Reading tempo breakdown

Now let me show you the breakdown and how tempo is to be read in a workout template. If someone writes for example

2:0:2:0 in a workout template, for instance, you are doing a push up this would mean that two seconds down would be the lowering portion or the eccentric, the second number would mean a pause at the bottom or in the middle the third would be the pushing up or the concentric portion of the repetition and the final would be at the top of the exercise. If there is a hold at the top or in the middle, it should be specified where the hold is in the middle or top/bottom. In a nutshell, this is how you would read a tempo. If the program has "x" in the tempo, it means lift as explosively in that lifting phase as you can.

Tempo breakdown for beginners.

For someone who is just beginning to workout, slower on the eccentric (on the way down) and a little bit faster on the concentric (on the way up), the reason why is so that we can start firing the right muscle fibers because in the beginning stage of working out people tend to compensate other muscles fiber which they use most often. Doing it slow something like 4:0:1:0 tempo would be a lot more beneficial for you.

How sets are used for different goals.

Sets are not so tricky as reps and tempo none the less, it is still important that they are used correctly towards your goal, now basic sets scheme is three sets, which can be used in a beginner/ intermediate lifter/ trainee who wants to put on some muscle. But if you're an advanced lifter three sets might be the thing of the past. Let us talk about how sets should be used for a beginner who is stepping in the gym for the first time. 1-2 sets per exercise with sufficient amount of break.

Do that for 2-4 weeks depending on how you feel, then you can slowly start doing two exercises in the same sets back to back. This will build more muscle endurance and give your muscle more time under tension. I would not recommend doing this if you are about to perform a big compound movement like bench press, squat or deadlift as the exercise itself is taxing enough and if you back to back it will only make your sets moving on weaker, especially if you're training for strength. Just focus on your main movements first and then for your accessory you can change back to back on exercises. If your goal is hypertrophy and you have been working towards the goal of putting on some muscle for about a year or so, then back to back sets can really be beneficial for someone who is training towards that.

Since it provides time under tension and you are able to add more exercises in your workout which equals more volume, that's major when it comes to hypertrophy for bodybuilding. For someone trying to get strong higher sets and lower reps would be the way to go so higher intensity meaning heavier weights and lower reps.

Primal movements

Most people workout because they want to put on muscle or they want to lose some fat, and some just want to work out to get in shape and live a healthier life. All the scenarios above need to be doing something called a primal movement. These movements all together workout your whole body in such a manner that these movements will not only help you get stronger or give you that aesthetic look that you're going for but this will also help you in day to day life hence known as a primal movement. Normally there are four primal movements, but personally, with years of experience in this field, I have decided to make it five primal movements, so here they are 1. Squat 2. Inverted rows/Trx rows (either works and can be adjusted to your physical capacity) 3 Push-ups/ modified push-ups 4. Hinge/ modified deadlift 5. Planks/ Abdominal work (depending on your fitness level).

All these primal movements can be modified to be accessible for anyone with any fitness level. Let's just say you cannot do push-ups off the floor. What you can do to make this movement more accessible to you is by doing it off your knees meaning instead of your toes you can use your knees as a pivot point or use a bench or a squat rack with a barbell and have your torso more upright or in an elevation which will make it easier for you to perform a push up. That goes with any primal movement all of them can be modified to fit your need, if primal movements are getting easy for you then we can also make it harder by adding some resistance and or elevating it.

Making an exercise easier is what we call a regression and making an exercise harder is what we call progression. It doesn't matter if you are really advanced or just merely a beginner, primal movements are to be performed to reach optimal results whether it be you living a healthier life or you just wanting to add that extra pound of muscle. These movements are a very important tool and should be used correctly for your individual needs and should be done safely. Now I will go thru all the primal changes with you and teach you the regression and progressions to these exercises.

Squat regression to progression

Let us start with regression if you cannot perform a bodyweight squat, what you start with is something called a box squat. Squat back like you are sitting back onto a chair and then with one second pause onto the box get back up into a standing position, a proper squat would be when your knees and your hips are below 90 degrees when you look at it from the side, if that's hard for you to achieve even with a box then start with a higher box or chair sit back on it and get back up and repeat that for sets and reps until it starts to feel like a 5 out of 10 in terms of how difficult it is. Then to progress from that do the same thing but lower the box or get a smaller chair. Keep doing that until you have managed to get below 90 degrees, now when going past 90 degrees on your box squats and it starts to feel easy then instead of pausing just tap the box and get back up instead of fully sitting on to the bench this will feel a lot harder, eventually when it starts to feel like a 5 out of 10 then you should be able to do bodyweight squats. If you can't then regress back to box squats with the tap and keep doing that until it feels like a 3 out of 10 and later tries out bodyweight squats.

Now when bodyweight squats start to feel like a 5 out of 10 then we can slowly begin to using some resistance to make it more challenging for you, one of the ways you can make this challenging is by performing something called a goblet squat basically what it is you hold a kettlebell or dumbbell, and you hold it up to your chest level with both of your hands, if this description doesn't explain the exercise properly there are a lot of videos online that will show you how to perform them in a detailed manner. If you don't have access to any kettlebell or dumbbell, then you can wear a backpack and you load the backpack up with some more substantial things laying around at your disposal, something like a heavy textbook or bottle of water. When you are capable of doing more than 45 lbs. of the kettlebell, dumbbell or any weight can be used on the squat for reps, then we can perhaps get into a safety bar squat or a barbell back squat, which one you move to depends on your shoulder mobility.

Rowing/Pull-ups Regression to Progression

Rowing is pretty easy to regress and progress from, the first thing you can start with is band rows or machine rows whatever you have available to you, start light and slowly up the resistance whether it be bands or machine rows. When you have managed to row about 3/4 of your bodyweight for 10 reps using machine rows or bands then you should be able to do an inverted rows, if you are using bands as resistance but you don't know what's the resistance is in pounds then get up to the most massive band you have and row that for 10 and later try inverted rows you should be able to get it done, beware there as bands with insane resistance, so don't take banded rows lightly. When you can do inverted rows, you should be closer to doing a pull-up, if you can complete a full

bodyweight pull up after that great if not here are a couple of things you can do.

If you have a pull up the assisted machine you can use that, start with a weight that you can do pull-ups with for 10 to 12 reps with and when it starts to feel like a 5 out of 10 then lower the weight so you get less resistance. Then repeat the same process until you can do a pull-up. Let's say don't have access to pull up assistance machine, what you can do is use bands to make it easier for you, just hang the group in the middle of the pull up bar or if you have a pull up bar with different grips then just hang it on to the handle that you aren't going to be using. Now from there get one of your knees onto the band and start doing pull-ups this will help you get some resistance from the band, which will make it easier for you to do a pull up, same principle applies as assisted pull up machine, go to a lighter band when it starts to feel like a 5 out of 10 at the end you should be able to do a pull up. Now let us just say you don't have access to bands or pull up assistance machine, in that case, you can do something known as eccentrics all you need to merely is get at the top of the pull up bar by using a chair or something elevated to get you to the top without any effort and from there slowly lower yourself and repeat the process, combine this with other back excises to strengthen your back and then you should be able to complete a pull up.

Push Ups Regression to Progression

Same as rows push-ups should be easy to regress and progress from if you can't do a push up off the floor here are a couple of things you can do to make it happen. If you have access to a squat rack and a barbell what you can do is merely do push-ups from an elevation meaning place the barbell on the latches that the squat rack has on them and then simply do push-ups from there so your torso is elevated which will make it easy for you to do push-ups, let's say you can do push-ups off number 13 on the squat rack riser keep doing that until it feels like a 5 out of 10 in terms of how hard it then lowers the latch and keep doing that until you can do a push up off the floor.

Now let us just say you don't have access to a squat rack just do push-ups off your knees and use that as your pivot point instead of your toes after when it feels like a 5 out of 10 then you should be able to do a push-up. If you can't even do push-ups off your knees what you can do is do more exercises that strengthen shoulders, triceps, and chest and then try doing push-ups off your knees you should be able to eventually.

Hinge/Deadlift

The main thing in deadlift/ hinge is not to squat the movement, instead, hinge it. I see a lot of people do this movement incorrectly for a lot of reasons, their lower back is rounding, or they are squatting the weight instead of performing a deadlift, there are a lot of other faulty movement patterns that can be causing poor form in the deadlift/hinge, but we will cover the basics. What does it mean to hinge instead of squatting, just put push your hips back , believe it or not a lot of people tend to have issues pushing their hips back and leaning your torso forward while keeping your back straight and it could be a lot of reasons, but one of them could be gluteus and hamstring tightness, which you should be working on in order to achieve a great deadlift/hinge. Now since we have gotten that covered first exercise which will progress us to a proper deadlift is kettlebell/ dumbbell and will be using a riser or a stool to which you will be touching your kettlebell/ dumbbell to as you are leaning your torso forward and pushing your hips back, meaning that the stool will be behind you and low enough for you to bend your torso forward while keeping your back flat, depending on your fitness and mobility level adjust the height of the riser/stool.

The best cue for a deadlift/hinge would be 1. stand up straight with a kettlebell or with dumbbell having your feet shoulder width apart or slightly wider whatever you feel comfortable doing 2. Bend your knees softly and have the pressure on the middle of your foot 3. Push your hips back while keeping your arms as close your body as possible and keeping the elbows straight not bent. 4. Touch the riser which is behind you. Start off like that and slowly lower the riser height to the point where you are touching the kettlebell/ dumbbell off the floor while keeping your back flat making sure you are pushing your hips back instead of squatting, and if you have issues keeping your back flat or you can't seem to bring the level down of your riser while keeping your back flat it could be your gluteus and hamstrings which are tight so look up some stretches on YouTube or google it, most of you should be able to progress to a lower riser or stool after that. After following the steps listed above, you should be ready to move into a Barbell/Trap bar deadlift.

Planks/Abdominal work

When you are performing the squats, push-ups, and rows you are using a lot of your core as these exercises require you to be stable throughout the movement, so in my opinion a lot of core/Abdominal training is needed, if you are performing abdominal exercises for aesthetic reasons planks might not be your go to. Now let us keep it simple if you have a big gut I would not recommend doing planks as it can put a lot of pressure on your lower back if you try and hold it for a more extended period of time.

When you perform push-ups you are working out your core, for someone with big gut push-ups is excellent for plank substitute, I would recommend doing something like crunches or leg raises instead and do your primal movements, and when you have managed to reduce your gut, you can go ahead and perform some planks. If you are on the chubbier side, you can do planks, but if you are on the side of being obese and your gut comes out a lot, that's when you shouldn't be performing planks, just wanted to clear that out. Now let's talk about progression and regression, if you are starting off and you do have a bigger gut start off with leg raises/ crunches either works, I would recommend more doing leg raises as it is easier on your spine, but either works just to make sure your spine is flat as you can keep it on your way up, start with 5 - 10 reps when it starts to feel like a 5 - 10 add extra 5 more reps so on and so forth. Now for planks , start off with however long you can hold a plank, let's say 30 seconds, when the 30 seconds starts feeling like a 5-10 go up to 45 seconds keep doing this until you can hold a plank for 2 minutes, after that is achieved add more weight to you back to make it harder.

Example workout plan

Exercise	Sets	Reps	Tempo
Push ups	3	10	4:0:2:0
Rows	3	10	4:0:2:0
Bodyweight squats	3	10	4:0:2:0
Hinge movement (any)	3	10	4:0:2:0

This would be one of the more basic workout plans, anyone can follow it. Make sure that you up to the intensity if you required by adding more supersets. Overall this workout is just an example, after reading this chapter you should have a very clear understanding of how to follow a workout plan and how to make one of your own based on your goals. Don't forget that it is very important for you to work out when following the alkaline diet, so make sure you get your workouts in however you want them.

Chapter 8: The 80/20 rule

Before we get into the 80/20 rule, I would like to talk about simple things when it comes to following the alkaline diet. When it comes to following the alkaline diet, there a lot of things to consider before you get into it. In fact, we haven't even touched upon the essential elements when it comes to following the alkaline diet, and we are going to touch upon that in this chapter right now. We will talk about how to start as a beginner and how to slowly scale up your diet in order to make sure that you are doing it correctly. Another thing is that many beginners will make a lot of newbie mistakes, which is why we need to talk about them and to help them understand how to avoid them in the long run. With that being said, let's talk about some of the things you need to take care of when following the alkaline diet.

Take a look at your diet

The alkaline diet works excellent, but it works a lot better when you eat healthier overall. For you to achieve better results from the Alkaline diet, it needs to be health-focused meals. You see when you start following the Alkaline diet alongside a healthy diet, and magic starts to happen. What we will do is give you great pointers on how to begin observing the Alkaline diet the right way.

We previously method before the macros and the eating patterns we recommended for people following the Alkaline diet, so let us recap them. If your goal is to lose some body fat your macros should be 40% protein 20% carbs and 40% fats, whereas if your goal is to maintain your weight and reap the benefits of Alkaline diet, then we recommend following a macro protocol of 30% protein 40% carbs and 30% fats. If you want to lose some weight, then you need to look at your diet, making sure you don't go over your calories and macros. If you aren't eating healthy meals throughout the day, then you can slowly start to incorporate better meals.

Start by having one healthy meal when you start your diet and one meal of whatever you desire, and once you become more comfortable, you can make it two meals, so on and so forth. Making you slowly start eating healthier, which will yield even better results overall. Yes, many people do get away with eating foods that aren't healthy, and yes, they so see unusual changes. However, if you want to see over the top health changes, then we recommend eating healthy and planned. Now there is no specific diet you need to follow other than the Alkaline diet, merely make healthier choices as this should help. You need to have a good look at your food, which you are eating and makes changes where necessary. It will be difficult in the start, but it will eventually become more natural.

Learn to listen to your body

It's essential that you understand to your body when you're dieting, listening to your body will help you understand when to stop and when not stop. Alkaline diet for women can require extra attention, and that is why it is necessary to listen to your body. There are some significant signs to look out for when following an Alkaline diet, know that most of the symptoms should subside in about a week.

However, if they don't chance are you need to switch up your dieting protocol. One of the ways to tell the Alkaline diet is becoming way too hard for you, is when you start feeling cold chronically. Once you begin to feel cold chronically, that's a big sign that Alkaline diet is becoming very hard for you to follow if you feel cold throughout the day for three weeks plus then chances are it is time for you to lower the dieting intensity. Another sign to consider when your Alkaline diet would be extreme hunger.

The first couple of weeks you will feel extreme hunger, but if that keeps happening for over three weeks chances are your body is telling you that you can't follow Alkaline diet at this level. These are the significant signs you need to listen to your body when Alkaline diet, but always make sure you get your blood work done and get the professional help if you feel like Alkaline diet is affecting you physically. Best rules to live by when Alkaline diet if it doesn't feel right three weeks into it then stop. Nonetheless, symptoms could occur anytime, just be in-tuned with your body and make sure you are listening to it.

Helpful tips dealing with hunger

When following an Alkaline diet routine, it is crucial that you make sure that your appetite is under control to make sure diet isn't broken prematurely. Time and time again, many followers of the Alkaline diet have broken the diet prematurely just because they couldn't control their hunger. We will go multiple ways to deal with desire, and overall help you continue with the Alkaline diet. The first tip is pretty obvious, and that is to drink more water. Much of the time, hunger is thirst.

Meaning you will be able to control your eating desires by drinking more water, having more water through the day helps you tremendously to control your hunger. Another method for managing your appetite would be to drink more green tea, and caffeine has shown to suppress, which overall helps you with dieting. Just make sure the tea you drink does not contain any sugar or milk, as that could break your diet. Getting yourself busy will help you control your hunger. Most of the time, when we occupy yourself with work, we tend to forget the food.

Perhaps do some work, or household chores to keep yourself busy when you feel like eating. You can also exercise or go for a walk, and this will kill two birds with one stone. When you start walking, you will take your mind of dieting, and you will also burn some fat while doing so. If you are feeling more energetic, then you can go ahead and get a full workout. However, remember that you might feel hungry after the exercise if you have no experience in managing your hunger. Now, if you are looking for a more relaxed way of handling your appetite, then we would recommend meditation.

Meditation works well when it comes to controlling your hunger, and it will also help you manage your mental stress if you have any. Make sure you are using this tool, to manage your appetite, and who knows you might really enjoy meditation. The final technique we recommend would be to eat more fibrous foods when dieting, as this will help you stay fuller for an extended period. Many followers of the Alkaline diet will eat anything Alkaline, and this will actually make them crave foods faster than someone who ate a good healthy meal with a ton of fiber in it.

If you want to have a better, less hungry dieting window, then we highly recommend you eat healthy meals with a ton of fiber in them during your diet. These are all the tips and tricks to dealing with hunger, make sure that you are following all these tips to control your appetite when dieting. Especially if it is your first three weeks dieting, as that is when you will notice most of the hunger cravings. These tips will help you tremendously to power through those first three weeks, and help you with completing your diet.

80/20 rule

Since you now have understood the basics of the alkaline diet, let's talk about the 80/20 rule and how it can help you tremendously when it comes to following the alkaline diet and to make your lifestyle a lot easier. As we previously mentioned to you, whenever you're eating any kind of protein, you will be increasing your acidic levels in the body. Which is inevitable when it comes to following the alkaline diet, as you might know, you cannot be alkaline all the time which is why it is essential that you take care of yourself properly and to use this diet and the right way when it comes to putting on muscle or whatever your goal is.

Simply put it, alkaline diet and the 80/20 rule goes hand-in-hand when it comes to making a lifestyle. The 80-20 rule simply means that 80% of your food is going to be alkaline, and 20% of the food can be acidic. Also, many people say that the 80/20 rule is the ideal way to go about following the alkaline diet as a keeps you healthy overall. Many people staying alkaline every time all the time can be unhealthy, which is why it is essential that you include the 80/20 rule in your diet when following the alkaline diet. Now the only reason why the 80/20 rule works is that you're going to be a plant-based eater. If you are going to be eating meat, then there's a high chance that you're going to be a lot more acidic than the 80/20 rule. Which is why we highly recommend that you start following a plant-based diet when it comes to following the alkaline diet and to see the best results overall.

Other things you also need to understand when following the alkaline diet, is that every food that we're going to be eating is metabolized and leaves behind ash which is why sometimes the alkaline diet is called the alkaline Ash diet. This ash will either alkaline-forming or acidic forming. As you know, when you are giving your body consistently acidic foods, it will cause it to become a lot more vulnerable to illness and diseases like high blood pressure cholesterol heart diseases and even cancer. As we told you, it is much better to be in a higher alkaline level in the body. However, you're inevitably going to be alkaline for the rest of your life, as the waste you're going to be reducing from your bodies like your urine and other things will be a lot more acidic which is why it is essential that you understand that and go along with it. Overall, we have understood that acidic diets can be awful for us.

Which is why we need to make a change in our diet, many people think that following the alkaline diet is the right way to go about it and will go full out on the alkaline diet disregarding any acidic meals. Although this might work for you in the short-term, this will not be feasible for you in the long term once you start to really follow the diet. The thing is, it is impossible for us to avoid any of the acidic foods. Which is why it is imperative that we have some of this set of foods in our diet, helping us not go crazy and to see the best benefits overall. Which is when the 80-20 rule comes in, the 80/20 rule allows you to eat 20% of the foods and acidic level and 80% of the basic level.

This will give you a great balance when it comes to following this diet and will also help you to stop and give up the cravings that you might be facing when following the alkaline diet. If you don't know, many of the yummy foods that we're going to be eating are going to come from acidic foods. Which makes it insanely impossible for us to be 100% alkaline all the time. Following the 80/20 rule will also give you a leeway when it comes to living your lifestyle overall, here's the thing if you go to you are at your friend's birthday party what are the chances that you are actually going to be eating some cake and drinking some alcohol.

The chances are very high, which is why we recommend that you follow the 80/20 rule which will allow you to eat a little bit more food what you might like and to combat it if you overeat. If you know that you're going to your friend's birthday party, then make sure that you eat very alkaline until the lead-up off his birthday. This will allow you to keep your body very alkaline, and then to indulge in some acidic foods that will enable you to keep the 80/20 rule rolling and therefore helping you be better and happy life overall. Here's the thing, it is impossible to follow a diet once it becomes a chore. And if you are trying to follow a 100% alkaline diet, not only is it going to be unhealthy for you and will also cause a lot of issues when it comes to long-term effects of it, which is why we highly recommend when following the alkaline diet with the use of the 80/20 rule. This will allow you to enjoy your life a lot better and to see the benefits of the alkaline diet, and the alkaline diet will only work if you do it in the long-term process, which means that you need to follow the alkaline diet for a very long time before you start seeing the results. Remember, it is a more lifestyle than it is more a diet. Another way to make sure that you stay alkaline throughout the whole day is to make sure that you are drinking alkaline water and also that you are working out.

Many people think that if they follow the alkaline diet, it is ok not to work out, which is not the case. The thing is that working out is one of the best things you can do for your health and overall wellness. When accompanied alkaline diet with a good workout, then you will notice one of the best results when it comes to putting on muscle and looking a lot better. Whether your goals to lose fat put on muscle or just to look better overall, you need to make sure that you're incorporating a good workout plan with your alkaline diet to see the best results possible. Any training plan will work, as long as it has been created by a professional and that it is accustomed to your needs. The great thing about the 80/20 rule is that it can be combated if you start working out.

When you work out, your body will become a lot more alkaline and therefore help you combat any issues that you might be facing and thus help you put on more muscle more specifically make you more alkaline throughout the whole day. It is essential that you work out with your 80/20 rule, as some days you might be over 20% of acidic level but you can combat it with the use of workouts. With that being said, I hope they've understood how to use the 80/20 rule properly and how to use the alkaline diet overall. After reading all these chapters, you should have an excellent idea on how to follow the alkaline diet, if not make you a mini-expert on it. With that being said, let us give you an example of a seven-day meal plan, which will allow you to come up with your own menu making the alkaline diet an easy diet to follow.

7-day eating plan

Example meal plan:

Monday

Breakfast - Wild rice cream of rice, almond milk, and berries

Snack - Green tea

Lunch - Salad with balsamic vinegar

Snack - Wild grain pita bread with hummus

Dinner - Plant-based meat substitute (found at a grocery store), cherry tomatoes and arugula.

Tuesday

Breakfast - Whole wheat pancakes or pancakes made from oats powders, served with berries and raw honey

Snack - nuts and berries

Lunch -sprouted beans and Greek salad

Snack - Almond butter, on wild grain bread

Dinner - wild rice with beans boiled veggies (broccoli, asparagus, and spinach)

Wednesday

Breakfast - egg substitute (in recipes chapter) with toast (whole wheat)

Snack - Smoothie with fruits and veggies

Lunch - Salad with beans and vegetables

Snack - vegan protein

Dinner - Tofu Squeers (with your favorite herbs or spices) with wild rice and veggies

Thursday

Breakfast - Fresh veggie/fruit smoothie

Snack - Handful of trail mix

Lunch - sprouted beans with boiled veggies and balsamic vinegar

Snack - Fruits

Dinner - lentils and red onion with a dressing of extra-virgin olive oil with your favorite seasoning

Friday

Breakfast - Low sugar cereal almond milk and berries

Snack - green tea

Lunch - Salad with balsamic vinegar

Snack - Pita bread with hummus

Dinner - Whole wheat bread with eggs substitute (in the recipes section) cherry tomatoes and arugula.

Saturday

Breakfast - Wild rice cream of rice, with almond milk

Snack - Healthy smoothie

Lunch - vegan protein shake with fruits

Snack - Almonds hand full

Dinner -Alkaline beans wild rice and a side of veggies and extra virgin olive oil.

Sunday

Breakfast - Whole wheat pancakes or pancakes made from oats powders, served with berries and raw honey

Snack - Vegan protein with fruits

Lunch - vegan meat substitute, Greek salad

Snack - Almond butter, on whole wheat bread

Dinner - sprouted with boiled veggies (broccoli, asparagus, and spinach)

As you can see, this chapter will help you to predispose your menu. The whole point is to make this diet very easy for you to follow, which was one of the goals of this chapter.

Chapter 9: Recipes

If switching to the alkaline diet feels a little overwhelming, a good place to start is to look at some of your current favorite recipes and see what ingredients you can substitute. Meat may feel like the biggest challenge, but below we list several vegan meat substitutes. Many of these provide the flavor and texture of meat you crave as well as plant-based proteins that are often lost when removing animal-based foods from your diet.

Tofu is a soy-based product that easily takes on the flavors of the other ingredients in the recipe. This Asian staple is high in protein and calcium and can easily be a substitute for beef, pork, chicken, or seafood. Tofu has a bad reputation for being bland and spongy, though extra-firm tofu can be implemented into any recipe after being pressed, which removes extra liquid. This brings the texture of tofu closer to a firm and chewy meat. When cooking with tofu, be sure to add extra spices and seasoning to the recipe, as tofu will absorb it and take in the flavor.

Textured Vegetable Protein, also known as TVP, is another soy-based product, only this is dehydrated, making it inexpensive and easy to store. Much like tofu, it absorbs any flavor you throw it in, only needing extra liquid to bring it back to life. TVP can be a substitute for recipes that call for ground meat such as meatloaf or burgers.

Jackfruit, a healthy tropical fruit, has become a recent top choice in meat replacement. It naturally has a meaty texture, though simply roasting it in the oven for about 15 minutes can help take it to the next level. From there, you can chop it, shred it, or leave it in a solid piece and add any flavoring you please. Jackfruit is often used as a pork substitute, though this tends to be a fun ingredient to experiment with.

Tempeh has a grainy texture and is firmer than extra-firm tofu. Also made from soy, this meat substitute has a nuttier flavor. Tempeh contains a healthy amount of protein, along with calcium, fiber, and vitamins. It is a little easier to handle than tofu because you don't need to press it. Rather, tempeh is very versatile that you can grind it, chop it, slice it, dice it—do whatever suits your recipe. Tempeh can have a bitter flavor, which can be remedied by steaming before using it. It is often used as a fish substitute, based on its particular texture.

Mushrooms give a lovely earthy flavor and come in many varieties. Large whole caps like those on portobello mushrooms can be used in one piece as a burger or a "plate" for stuffing other ingredients. They can also be thrown in the food processor for a filling meat substitute with softer texture like that of tenderized and slow cooked meats.

Lentils are an old favorite in the world of veganism. They are inexpensive, easy to store, come in a few different varieties, and can easily be boiled and ready in a short amount of time. Use lentils to substitute the ground beef in your recipes.

Some "honorable mention" ingredients you may want to consider stocking up on include cauliflower, beans and legumes, beets, eggplant, potatoes, and coconut. These are ingredients that replace meat as well as grain-based food if gluten is a concern.

I know some of these foods could be considered acidic, however, if you read the chapter where we talked about the 80/20 rule then you should have no problem with having some acidic foods here and there. It is essentially impossible to have a fully alkaline diet. Regardless, here are some amazing recipes which you could follow to help your cravings and to see better results with your alkaline diet.

Chickpea Omelet

Taking out eggs from your diet may be one of the most significant breakfast challenges you will come across. This unique recipe can be made with any toppings you would like to start your day. Recommended toppings include sautéed mushrooms, tomatoes, green peppers, and onion.

Ingredients:
- One cup chickpea flour
- Half teaspoon onion powder
- one-third cup nutritional yeast

- half teaspoon baking soda
- one-fourth teaspoon black pepper
- one-fourth teaspoon white pepper
- half teaspoon garlic powder
- One cup of water

Chocolate Pancakes

Everyone deserves chocolate for breakfast every once in a while. Satisfy your sweet tooth with these gluten-free, vegan chocolate pancakes that go well with almost any fruit of choice, especially strawberries, bananas, and raspberries.

Ingredients:
- One ¼ cup gluten-free flour of choice
- One tablespoon ground flaxseed
- One tablespoon baking powder
- Three tablespoons nutritional yeast
- Two tablespoons unsweetened cocoa powder
- ¼ teaspoon of sea salt
- 1 cup unsweetened, unflavored almond milk
- One tablespoon vegan mini chocolate chips (optional)

- One teaspoon vanilla extract
- ¼ teaspoon stevia powder or 1 tablespoon pure maple syrup
- One tablespoon apple cider vinegar
- ¼ cup unsweetened applesauce.

Instructions:

Get a medium sized bowl and mix all the dry ingredients (flour, baking powder, flaxseed, cocoa powder, yeast, salt, and optional chocolate chips). Whisk until evenly combined.

In a different small bowl, combine wet ingredients except for the applesauce (almond milk, vanilla extract, apple cider vinegar, maple syrup or stevia powder).

Add wet ingredient mixture and applesauce to the dry ingredients and mix by hand until ingredients are just combined.

The batter should sit for 10 minutes. It will rise and thicken, possibly doubling in size.

Heat an electric griddle or nonstick skillet to medium heat and spray with a small amount of nonstick spray, if desired — scoop batter into 3-inch rounds. Much like traditional pancakes, bubbles will start to appear. When bubbles begin to burst, flip pancakes and cook for 1-2 minutes. Yields 12 pancakes.

Breakfast Scramble

Here is another egg-free breakfast option for the veggie lover! Many scramble recipes call for tofu, whereas here we are using cauliflower. This recipe is unique and allows you to use whichever veggies you may already have in your refrigerator. Feel free to substitute at will!

Ingredients:

- One large head cauliflower cut up
- One seeded, diced green bell pepper
- One seeded, diced red bell pepper
- 2 cups sliced mushrooms (approximately 8 oz whole mushrooms)
- One peeled, diced red onion
- Three peeled, minced cloves of garlic
- Sea salt
- 1 ½ teaspoons turmeric

- 1–2 tablespoons of low-sodium soy sauce
- ¼ cup nutritional yeast (optional)
- ½ teaspoon black pepper

Instructions:

1. Sauté green and red peppers, mushrooms, and onion in a medium saucepan or skillet over medium-high heat until onion is translucent (should be 7–8 min). Add an occasional tablespoon or two of water to the pan to prevent vegetables from sticking.

2. Add cauliflower and cook until florets are tenders. Should be 5 to 6 minutes.

3. Add, pepper, garlic, soy sauce, turmeric, and yeast (if using) to the pan and cook for about 5 minutes.

Superfood Breakfast Bars

Need a quick pre-made breakfast option you can grab and go? This breakfast bar is not only sweet and salty, but it's also vegan, gluten-free, and packed with superfood energy.

Ingredients:

- Four apples

- 1.5 cups mix of mulberries and goji berries, soaked in lukewarm water for about 30 minutes
- 1 cup all-natural apple juice + 3 tablespoons divided
- Two tablespoons maple syrup
- 2-3 tablespoons sunflower seed butter
- Two teaspoons aluminum free baking powder
- 4 cups gluten-free certified oats
- Pinch of cinnamon (optional)
- Sunflower seeds for garnish

Instructions:

1. Preheat your oven to 390 degrees Fahrenheit.

2. Line the 11" x 8" baking dish with parchment paper.

3. Chop apples coarsely and remove seeds. Add to blender with one c. of the apple juice. Blend until smooth

4. Mix the remaining three tablespoons of apple juice, sunflower butter, and maple syrup in a small bowl. You will create a creamy and smooth paste.

5. In a large bowl, combine the soaked and trained berries, oats, sunflower paste, baking powder, and apple mix into a well-mixed dough.

6. Press the dough with a spatula or your hands in the baking dish. Top it with sunflower seeds. Bake for 20 min.

Mac and Cheese Bites

Welcome to the vegan twist on an old classic. We promised this book would help satisfy some of your past, pre-vegan cravings, so here's a great portable comfort food bite that will please kids and grown-ups alike. Note that these can be eaten warm or cold, though warming them up may make them fall apart a bit.

Ingredients:
- 1 ½ cups uncooked macaroni (gluten-free will work if needed)
- One medium onion, chopped (can substitute with one medium yellow pepper if you don't care for onions.)
- One clove garlic, chopped
- Two tablespoons cornstarch, or arrowroot powder
- 1 cup non-dairy milk
- ½ teaspoon smoked paprika (can substitute for chipotle powder)
- One teaspoon lemon juice or apple cider vinegar

- ½ cup nutritional yeast
- One teaspoon salt

Instructions:

1. Preheat your oven to 350 degrees Fahrenheit.

2. Prepare the muffin tin with liners.

3. Prepare macaroni according to instructions.

4. While macaroni is cooking, sauté garlic and onion (or substitute of choice) until it is just starting to turn golden brown. This can be done in a dry pan, but adding some oil will work as well.

5. Add garlic, onion, and all other non-macaroni ingredients into a blender and mix until smooth.

6. Drain the macaroni and return to the pan.

7. Pour sauce over macaroni and stir well.

8. Spoon mixture into muffin tin, occasionally stirring in between such an equal amount of sauce goes in each cup.

9. Push down the top with the back of a spoon.

10. Bake in the oven for 30 min.

11. Serve once cooled.

Guacamole Stuffed Rolls

If you're seeking plant-based meals for weight loss, you may want to skip to the next recipe. This creamy, indulgent treat is based on the Hungarian cheese rolls, using puff pastries as a shell for your stuffing.

Ingredients:

- One sheet vegan puff pastry
- Two tablespoons almond milk (or other plant milk)
- One pinch turmeric

For the filling:

- One zucchini
- Juice of 1 whole lemon
- 2/3 cup raw cashews, soaked
- Two cloves of garlic
- One avocado, diced
- One teaspoon fresh, chopped chili pepper
- Two scallions
- One tablespoon chive, chopped

Instructions:

1. Cut puff pastry into eight strips. Roll each piece on a cream horn mold or some similar shape.

2. Bake rolls at 400° F for 20-25 min. Cool completely, then remove shells.

3. While rolls are baking, add zucchini, cashews, garlic, and lemon juice to blender or food processor. Blend until completely smooth. This will take some time. Once the mixture is smooth and creamy, add avocado, chili pepper, scallions, and chives, along with salt and pepper. Pulse a few times. 4. Pour mixture into a piping bag and fill puff pastry rolls.

Vegan Philly Cheesesteak

A great twist on a local favorite, this sandwich is reasonably simple to put together and contains ingredients that are easy to find. Can be served with vegan mayo, if desired.

Ingredients:

- 6-8 sliced Portobello mushrooms
- Four cloves garlic, minced
- One tablespoon olive oil

- One whole clove garlic
- ½ teaspoon black pepper
- One teaspoon dried thyme
- ½ large diced onion
- A dash of kosher salt
- One tablespoon vegan Worcestershire sauce
- Hoagie rolls or another small loaf of bread of choice
- 1 cup shredded vegan cheddar cheese
- Vegan mayo (optional)

Instructions:

1. Preheat the broiler.

2. In a deep skillet, heat olive oil. Brown mushrooms in oil, about 10 min.

3. Add thyme, garlic, and pepper until evenly coated.

4. Add onion and salt. Mushrooms must be well cooked before adding salt. Cook until onion is caramelized and softened, which should be for about 5 minutes. Add Worcestershire sauce and mix well.

5. Slice the bread lengthwise. Coat open sides of bread with olive oil or cooking spray. To add garlic flavor, cut whole

garlic clove, cut off the tip, and put on the oiled side of bread. Garlic powder is also a good substitute.

6. If desired, add optional vegan mayo. Place bread on cookie sheet. Fill loaves with mushrooms and top with shredded vegan cheddar cheese.
7. Place in broiler until cheese has melted, which should be 4-5 minutes.

Mango Lime Chia Pudding

Chia pudding is another versatile treat that can be used at breakfast or as a mid-day snack. Pack it in a mason jar or a recycled food jar. This is one of many flavor combinations you can create.

Ingredients:
- 3 cups fresh or frozen mango chunks
- One 15.5-ounce can coconut milk
- One tablespoon lime zest
- ¼ cup maple syrup
- ¼ cup freshly squeezed lime juice
- ¼ cup hemp seeds

- 1/3 cup chia seeds

Topping options: Approximately 8 cups of any combination of mango, banana, pineapple, or any fruit you'd love with mango and lime. (Banana is a fruit you'd want to wait to add until you are ready to eat the pudding as it browns and gets mushy very quickly once out of its peel)

Instructions:

1. Place mango chunks, coconut milk, lime zest, and maple syrup in a blender. Mix until smooth.
2. Add hemp and chia seeds in the blender and stir by hand or blend on low to just combine.
3. This should yield 4 cups of pudding. Portion it as you prefer. One suggestion is to divide into eight portions, one each in a pint jar, and top with one cup of fresh fruit.
4. Refrigerate pudding until ready to eat, minimum 4 hours to set. The pudding keeps for 5-7 days.

Mint Chocolate Truffle Larabar Bites

This copycat recipe can be rolled into individual balls or placed in a pan and cut up as bars after firming in the refrigerator. With 15-minute prep time, this quick fix will satisfy any sweet tooth! Can keep for three weeks if refrigerated in an airtight container.

Ingredients:

- 1 cup vegan chocolate chips (semi-sweet dark chips are recommended)
- Ten large Medjool dates
- 1 ½ cups of raw almonds
- ¼ cup coconut flour
- A ¼ cup of cocoa powder
- ¼-1/2 teaspoon peppermint extract
- Two tablespoons water

Instructions:

1. Pour almonds into a food processor and chop until a fine flour.

2. Add chocolate chips, dates, flour and cocoa, and process again until well combined.

3. Add oil and peppermint extract.

4. Process one more time until the mix starts balling up.

5. Taste a small bit and add more peppermint if you wish. Process again if you do.

6. Remove the blade from processor and form the dough into balls. Choose whatever size you like, as they do not need to bake and will be right in any portion.

Peanut Butter Caramel Rice Krispies

Take a trip down memory lane and bring the wonderful memory of rice krispie treats into the adult world. This healthier version will give you a light and crunchy snack that is great for munching at home or family potlucks.

Ingredients:
- 6 cups crisp rice cereal
- 1/3 cup creamy peanut butter (can substitute with almond or sunflower seed butter)
- ¾ cup brown rice syrup
- One teaspoon vanilla extract
- ¼ cup maple syrup

Peanut butter drizzle:

- Two tablespoons creamy peanut butter (or substitute of choice)
- One teaspoon maple syrup (or another liquid sweetener)
- 1-2 teaspoons to thin, if needed

Instructions:

1. Line a 9" x 9" square pan with parchment or wax paper. An 8" x 8" pan will work as well. Treats will just be thicker.

2. Place a large pot over medium heat. Add brown rice syrup and maple syrup in and bring to a rolling boil. Cook for 1-2 minutes, stirring often and making sure mix does not burn.

3. Remove from heat. Mix in vanilla and peanut butter with whisk until smooth.

4. In a large bowl, pour in crisp rice cereal. Stir in the liquid mix until well combined.

5. Scoop into pan and spread out evenly. Press down with wet fingers or spatula. Place in freezer to set for ten minutes while making peanut butter drizzle.

6. In a separate microwavable bowl, mix peanut butter and maple syrup. Microwave in 30-second intervals until just

warm for easier mixing. Add one teaspoon water at a time if needed. Mix until smooth.

7. Remove treats from freezer and drizzle on peanut butter mix. Place back in the fridge until firm ideally 10 min.

8. Cut into squares for serving. Bars will hold their shape very well at room temperature but can be stored in the fridge. Leftovers can be wrapped up and kept in the refrigerator for 5 to 7 days or freezer for up to one month.

Easy Chocolate Pudding

Get ready to throw away the instant boxed stuff and try this equally easy, dairy-free chocolate pudding that is so rich, creamy, and chocolatey that you won't believe that it's healthy and refined sugar-free. Top with some coconut whipped cream for a perfect treat.

Ingredients:

- 1 ½ cups organic coconut cream from a can
- ½ cup raw cacao powder (sifted unsweetened cocoa powder works as well)
- Six tablespoons pure maple syrup (may adjust to up to 8 tablespoons, depending on how sweet you like it)

- Two teaspoons pure vanilla extract
- Fine grain sea salt

Instructions:

1. In a small pan over low heat, whisk coconut cream, cacao, and maple syrup until smooth. A smaller whisk I make a more harmonious mixture. Continue to cook over low/medium for 2 minutes, or until the mixture starts to come to a boil with small bubbles.

2. Remove from heat. Add salt and vanilla. Stir. Taste and add more maple if you'd like a sweeter pudding. 3. Pour into individual containers/bowls or keep in one larger bowl to set.

4. Cover and refrigerate it until set, or overnight for a thick and creamy pudding. Makes four servings.

As you can see, we gave you some of the most amazing recipes which you can start following today. Keep in mind that our goal was to make the alkaline diet as fun as possible, which is why we added these unique recipes to this book.

Conclusion

Thank you so much for purchasing Alkaline diet for beginners the complete guide to understanding alkaline diet. Start the perfect meal plan to heal your body and eat well for weight loss. As you can tell, we talked about many things in this book, we covered most of the premises in regards to an alkaline diet and what it can do for you.

The alkaline diet is the diet you need to be following if your goal is to better your health or to live a healthy life. After reading this book, you can tell the importance of alkalinity and how it can help you to get rid of many diseases as well. Keep in mind, that you need to be physically active for the alkaline diet to work even better, which is why we included a workout plan and some pointers that will help you to create your workout routine.

Nonetheless, the alkaline diet will work for you if your goal is to put on muscle, lose weight, or get rid of diseases. This book is probably one of the most well-written books on the topic, and I'm sure you can agree with us after reading this book. With that being said, we conclude, thank you so much for reading till the end as it means a lot to us. As always, if you liked what you read, then make sure to leave us a good review on this book as it is essential for others to see how well this book has been written.

www.ingramcontent.com/pod-product-compliance
Lightning Source LLC
Chambersburg PA
CBHW060519290526
45791CB00001B/451